Planning in Health Promotion Work

An empowerment model

Roar Amdam

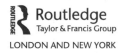

Routledge
Taylor & Francis Group

LONDON AND NEW YORK

First published 2011 by Routledge
2 Park Square, Milton Park, Abingdon, Oxfordshire OX14 4RN

Simultaneously published in the USA and Canada
by Routledge
711 Third Avenue, New York, NY 10017

*Routledge is an imprint of the Taylor & Francis Group,
an informa business*

First issued in paperback 2012

© 2011 Roar Amdam

Typeset in Sabon by
Florence Production Ltd, Stoodleigh, Devon

British Library Cataloguing in Publication Data
A catalogue record for this book is available
from the British Library

Library of Congress Cataloging-in-Publication Data
Amdam, Roar, 1951–
  Planning in health promotion work: an empowerment model/
  Roar Amdam.
      p. cm.
    Includes bibliographical references and indexes.
  1. Health planning.   2. Health promotion.   3. Regional medical
  programs.   4. Health planning—Baltic Sea Region.   5. Health
  promotion—Baltic Sea Region.   6. Regional medical programs
  —Baltic Sea Region.   7. HEPRO (Project) I. Title.
  [DNLM: 1. Regional Health Planning—methods—Europe.
  2. Consumer Participation—methods—Europe.   3. Health
  Promotion—methods—Europe.   4. Public Health Practice—
  Europe.   5. Public Policy Europe.   WA 541 GA1 A497p 2001]
  RA394.9.A43 2011
  362.1—dc22   2010012109

ISBN 13: 978-0-415-58367-1 (hbk)
ISBN 13: 978-0-415-82005-9 (pbk)
ISBN 13: 978-0-203-84252-2 (ebk)

Contents

Figures

Preface

Public health work is increasingly becoming a multi-sector and multilevel responsibility, and there is a need for a comprehensive community and regional planning approach. The HEPRO project was an example of this type of approach. According to the HEPRO project plan (Østfold County Council, 2005), the aim of the project was to integrate health considerations into spatial planning and development, and to make an important contribution to a sustainable public health policy in Europe. HEPRO consisted of thirty-two partners and brought together lay people and experts with specialist knowledge and experience from all relevant sectors across eight countries around the Baltic Sea Region (BSR; see the Appendix). The project's aim was to help to share effective ways to promote health and bring the results to the attention of those who needed to take action. The project was to carry out a transnational population survey and a training programme, and implement concrete findings from the survey into the spatial planning processes. The results were to be gathered in a toolkit, with the purpose to support decision-makers at regional and local level with evidence-based and practical advice. HEPRO was an EU–INTERREG III B project. The project period was from 1 June 2005 to 31 December 2007 (31 months). HEPRO had a budget of about €2 million.

I was invited into the HEPRO project to participate in public health planning as a planning expert, adviser and action researcher. In this situation, it became natural for me to summarize the knowledge and experiences we have from local and regional planning and development, and reflect on how to use this in public health planning. In accordance with the main goal of the HEPRO project, my role in the project became to develop and implement training programmes in public health work aimed at various target groups in order to build understanding of spatial health planning and the use of local health profiles.

Therefore, this book is based on my long-term work as a planner and researcher in the field of local and regional planning and development, combined with experiences from the HEPRO project and reflections on how this research can be adapted to public health planning. For me, individual and collective empowerment has been an overall driving force in this work.

I will say that the HEPRO project, as it was planned, could easily become a public health intervention with a bias towards top-down implementation, but, through the process and the emphasis on an empowerment planning approach, it became a more balanced, top-down and bottom-up project. One of the missions of this book is to introduce the empowerment planning approach used in the HEPRO project, and discuss this approach as a general planning model in public health work.

In the first chapter, I discuss how the HEPRO-project approach can be interpreted in a planning perspective, and I point out some of the main challenges the project is facing. In the second chapter, I discuss what can be called the governance turn in planning. This turn has a great impact on how we regard the role of the public sector, and how we can design the planning process. Then, in the third chapter, I discuss the theoretical foundation of the planning model used in the HEPRO project, and outline the empowerment planning model. In the fourth chapter, I discuss empowerment evaluation, and show how monitoring and evaluation can contribute to learning at different levels in the empowerment planning model. The last chapter is a summary of the previous chapters and reflects on the activities implemented by the partners during the project period.

I am grateful to many people who have contributed to the work for this book. First of all, I am grateful to the public health staff at Østfold County Council, and especially to the HEPRO project leader, Arvid Wangberg, and the head of the public health unit, Knut Johan Rognlien, who invited me to join this very interesting and demanding project, and to Tiina Keinänen for the work she did as project secretary. Then, I am very grateful to all the dedicated public health workers in the BSR who participated in the project. I am very honoured by the opportunity I got to work with all of you.

Roar Amdam, Volda

1   Perspectives on the HEPRO project approach

In this chapter, I present the HEPRO project, and discuss some perspectives that can place this project in the theoretical field and that can contribute to better understanding of the challenges the project is facing in practice.

The HEPRO project

The HEPRO project consisted of thirty-two partners and brought together lay people and experts with specialist knowledge and experience from all relevant sectors across eight countries around the BSR. The project was a part of the 'Healthy Cities' approach, a concept that is underpinned by the principles of the 'Health for all' strategy and 'Local agenda 21'. Strong emphasis was given to empowerment, including equity, participatory governance and solidarity, inter-sectoral collaborations, and actions to address the determinants of health. HEPRO was, further, a project the aim of which was to integrate health considerations into spatial planning and development, and to make an important contribution to a sustainable public health policy in Europe. The project aimed to put health high on the political and social agendas of cities, and to build a strong movement for public health at the local level in the BSR. The main objectives were (Østfold County Council, 2005: 5):

- to integrate health considerations into spatial planning and development;
- to show how health profiles and environmental factors related to health can be used as a basis for a sustainable public health policy at local and regional levels;
- to describe and test active elements in a sustainable public health policy based on spatial health planning;
- to carry out a survey of the population's state of health, where data can be used across national boundaries;
- to develop and implement training programmes in public health work aimed at various target groups, in order to build understanding of spatial health planning and the use of local health profiles; and

- to raise awareness of European cohesion strategies, and enhance understanding in rural districts and smaller towns of opportunities and challenges within the European community.

According to the HEPRO project plan, the BSR is facing enormous challenges related to an ageing population, migration of young people from rural areas to the cities, unemployment, increases in alcohol and drug abuse, and mental illness. An increasing part played by lifestyle diseases and injuries from accidents makes great demands on the future treatment capacity of the health services. The problems require imaginative, complex and diverse solutions. To do something about it will require the involvement and co-operation of many different sectors of society, local, regional and national authorities, and the general public. A solution must have as its focus, not only risk factors, which have to be removed to avoid damage, but also factors that are positive and promote health conditions for individuals. A mobilization of resources in a joint effort between the population and the public authorities is the best starting point for good regional and local solutions. The project therefore put into practice democracy and should involve a high degree of participation by the public in the decisions affecting their lives, health and well-being (Østfold County Council, 2005).

A major aim of the HEPRO project was to integrate health considerations into spatial planning and development and to make an important contribution to a sustainable public health policy in Europe. The project aimed to help the sharing of effective ways to promote health and bring the results to the attention of those who need to take action. The project was to carry out a transnational population survey and training programmes, and implement concrete findings from the survey into the spatial planning processes. The data from this survey have now been analysed and published (Rasmussen and Wangberg, 2009).

The spatial dimension was important in the project because society and the environment were seen in a context of rural towns, cities, and district and regional levels. Providing a focus for inter-sectoral planning and inter-sectoral action, the project established partnerships across national borders – a co-operation that was intended to increase the living conditions of the population in the BSR. The results were to be gathered in a *toolkit* that could support decision-makers at regional and local levels with evidence-based and practical advice (Østfold County Council, 2005). The toolkit has now been published (see Wangberg and Dyrseth, 2008).

As we understand the HEPRO project, the approach is characterized by:

1   a circular understanding of planning;
2   a system theoretical approach to policy production; and
3   a spatial and cross-sectoral focus on public health.

Circular understanding of the planning process

The HEPRO project was intended to use planning as a tool in the policy-making process, and, in accordance with the understanding of policy-making as an ongoing process, planning is understood as a circular process (see Figure 1.1). This planning circle was adapted to fit the HEPRO project from a much-used model in health promotion and health planning. According to Østfold County Council (2005), the HEPRO planning model represents a systematic and comprehensive, long-term approach to public health planning in communities, and the model is a systematic approach in six steps, linked together in a circle with a dynamic character. The circle follows a planning period of 4 years. The aim is to show, step by step, how a plan where health and well-being aspects are highlighted can be carried out and embedded in the ordinary planning of the municipality/county/district.

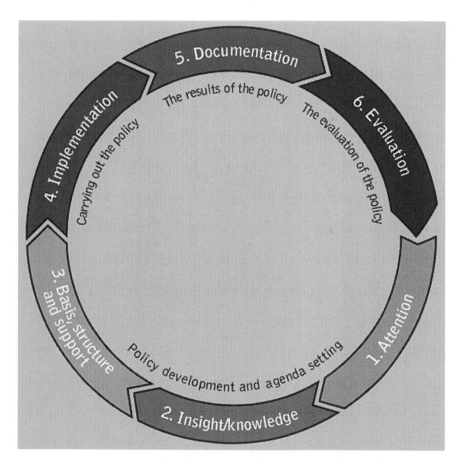

Figure 1.1 HEPRO planning circle
Source: Wangberg and Dyrseth (2008: 8)

The project presents the different stages of the circular process as follows (Wangberg and Dyrseth, 2008: 9):

1   *Attention*: Mapping the situation has an impact on the public health work through an analysis of strength, weakness, opportunities and threats (SWOT).
2   *Insight and new knowledge*: Mapping the situation gives new insight about local matters through a survey.
3   *Building a platform for joint action*: Based on insight and knowledge from steps 1 and 2, the project has to work out an action plan, and cross-sectoral workgroups must be established.
4   *Implementation*: Activities will be carried out in co-operation with local partners.
5   *Documentation*: Data from all activities that have been carried out must be collected in a systematic way as a basis for later evaluation.
6   *Evaluation*: The last step in the planning circle is an evaluation of structure, process and results. The results from the evaluation will give input to the starting point for a new planning circle.

Step 1: Attention – map the situation relevant to the public health effort

The project plan had, as a starting point, that public health work is not an issue for the public sector alone, but needs to involve the public, private and voluntary sectors, and national, regional and local governmental levels in a multi-actor approach, with the mission to promote good health and prevent bad health. The reason for this starting point was that public health work needs to convince the actors about the gains of the work and has to work with many actors in order to increase the capacity of implementation. Setting up an analysis of SWOT for the public health work in each partner community was an important part at this stage.

Our comment was that, compared with single public sectors such as culture, education, social care and health care, which all are well accepted and established in the political process and structure, public health work is cross-sector and cross-level work that has to fight for acceptances and build *legitimacy* in order to have impact on society. Legitimacy can be given to public health work, for example, when a community becomes a partner in an implementation structure such as HEPRO (top-down policy-making), or created through the mobilization and involvement of citizens in the work (bottom-up policy-making). In addition, legitimacy can be earned if the planning process is regarded as democratic, and people can observe an output and outcome of the process that they appreciate.

Step 2: Insight and new knowledge

The project plan stated that a *public health survey* is an important tool to map the public health situation in the different regions and districts.

The project plan argued for the health survey by stating that a survey gives a lot of different data about how people regard their situation, and what impact the public health work and other factors have on their situation. The data will be analysed and interpreted, and used in the planning and policy-making process. Actual problems will be sorted out, formulated and put on the political agenda.

Our comment is that this process can be very demanding. First of all, there is a need for expert competence to develop the survey, to analyse the collected data and to point out the major problems; then, there is a need for political skills to put these problems on the political agenda and to keep them there in competition with other political problems that must be solved. In addition, there is a need to involve lay people in dialogue between the experts and politicians, and to reach a common understanding of what problems need to be solved first and how people can contribute to solving the problems. The creation of this common understanding and the mobilization of people and their resources can increase the region's and district's capacity to handle the public health problems that are mapped in the survey. We said that the HEPRO project must understand the planning process as a *communicative process* involving persons from the public, private and voluntary sectors, and not as an *instrumental process*, with the planner as the expert and the most important person.

Step 3: Building a platform for joint action

According to the project plan, after putting public health on the political agenda at step 2, there follows step 3 and the need for organizing problem-solving activities. This is about creating action programmes, allocating budget resources, setting up cross-sectoral working groups, and involving the private and voluntary sectors in community development projects.

From our point of view, this step can become a battlefield between the power of vision and expectations and the power of resources and realism. The outcome of the battle is normally compromises, linked together in an incremental process where only small changes of direction can be obtained. However, small changes in the right direction can, over time, add up to big changes. So, in addition to organizing the big changes, is it important to have a clear focus on the small changes and to create a lasting platform for common actions. This means that setting up and deciding on a *public health action plan* can be an important event, but it is useless if the action plan is not implemented. To avoid this trap, our advice was to build structures and processes that constantly promote public health-friendly solutions and that remind people of the values of the public health work.

Step 4: Implementation

In the HEPRO planning circle, implementation is the fourth step. Our comments were that, in a linear way of thinking about planning, step 3 is followed by step 4. But it does not necessarily have to be like that because, in a society, there are always some activities that impact on people's health, and there will most certainly be some public, private or voluntary actors that continuously implement health promotion and prevention activities. The HEPRO project must therefore be understood as an intervention in a continuous public health work process, and the project must carry out activities in co-operation with local partners when they are ready to participate, and not wait with implementation of the activities until the action programmes are decided. In addition, relevant output from the project can contribute to the acceptance and legitimacy of the project, and the enforcement of public health work.

Step 5: Documentation

Documentation of the process and the activities is needed for the evaluation and learning process. To collect data about the process and the output is normally an easy part of this documentation. However, to get data about the outcomes and impacts, and then establish plausible causality between the input from the public health work and the impact on the public health situation, is a far more demanding and complicated task. Therefore, there seems, in a project such as this, to be a bias towards reporting the easily collected data about the output and neglecting the more difficult data about the outcomes. We warned that this situation could have consequences for the learning process, because there is a need for data about the impacts of the intervention in order to legitimate the public health work, keep it on the political agenda, involve more people and enforce the capacity to handle public health issues.

Step 6: Evaluation

The last step in the planning circle is an evaluation of structure, process and results. Evaluation will give input to the starting point for a new planning circle.

We argued that evaluation should be an integrated part of the whole process, and that reflection on the achieved results at every step of the circle could improve the capacity to handle the challenges in health promotion work. The SWOT analyses from step 1, the survey data from step 2, and experiences from creating the joint platform for action and implementation in steps 3 and 4 all represent data that are needed in the continuous evaluation of public health work. We will add here that, when the HEPRO project uses the circle as a metaphor, it is important to understand that, after one circuit, the participants in the process are not back where they started. The situation has changed, and the people involved have most certainly been learning, and new actions are taken up. Therefore, in our advice, we said that this model must be regarded as the main planning process, and that successful public health work needs to pay attention to all six steps at the same time over the whole period, because planning as policy-making is a continuous process. The different stages in the circle do not have to follow a fixed order. Implementation of one public health activity can go on simultaneously with efforts to generate attention and to put another activity on the political agenda.

When we compare the HEPRO planning model with other public health planning models and approaches, as described in McKenzie *et al.* (2005), it becomes clear that the HEPRO model, like many other models, is a combination of models. However, many of the models that are most used in practice and most thoroughly described in their book have a dominant, top-down programme implementation approach and regard the planning process as an instrumental activity with distinct steps or phases. Models such as PRECEDE-PROCEED, MATCH, CDCynergy and SMART represent a wide range of planning approaches; they share a common element in what can be called a *generalized model for programme planning*, with six steps in a linear process (McKenzie *et al.*, 2005: 16):

1   understanding and engaging
2   assessing needs
3   setting goals and objectives
4   developing an intervention
5   implementing the intervention
6   evaluating the result.

The 'Healthy community' or 'Healthy City' movement represents more communicative approaches to community planning and development than this generalized model. Although many of the steps associated with the 'Healthy community' approaches are quite similar to the generalized model, these approaches are characterized by health promotion and prevention as a continuous *capacity-building process* based on broad participation, communication, consensus building, empowerment, partnership, responsibility and community ownership. The HEPRO project is a part of the 'Healthy City' movement, and we regard the HEPRO planning model as an expression of the capacity-building planning approach associated with this movement.

We do not intend to go into a deeper discussion of policies, planning and strategies in health promotion here, but there are marvellous books about these topics. In addition to the already mentioned McKenzie *et al.* (2005), we can recommend Tones and Green (2004), Laverack (2005) and Green and Kreuter (2005).

The systemic approach to policy-making

Public health – a question about having political power

The HEPRO project regarded public health work as policy-making, and viewed the *policy process* in a system-theoretical perspective. The systemic approach to policy-making processes is well known from different authors and has been developed since Easton (1965), one of the first, used it. In the simplest form, the system model has an input, production and output element, and a feedback loop from the output to the input element. Pollitt and Bouckaert (2000) have a more elaborate contribution to the systemic approach, and their model focuses on important political and public issues (see Figure 1.2).

According to this model, political processes are illustrated by the left side representing the input for the decision process. The decision process is an arena where certain rules for how to make decisions can be introduced, and the right side of the model is the output of the decision process. The model illustrates the fact that actors outside the system of power, fighting for their values, interests and needs, can influence the structural power that, in time, has been integrated into the system of power (that is, presumptions, action patterns, routines, rules, and so on). In addition, the model highlights the

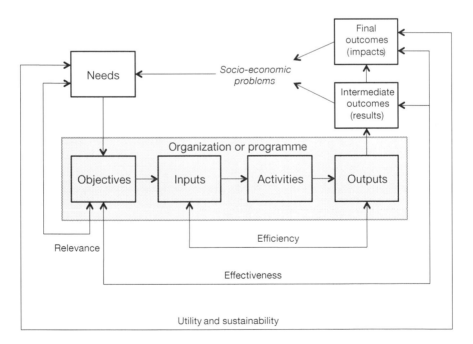

Figure 1.2 The policy process
Source: Pollitt and Bouckaert (2000: 106)

fact that the structural power can influence and socialize actors trying to achieve changes. Consequently, the model also gives an illustration of power not being a fixed variable, but subject to changes in both time and space.

The model also illustrates the different dimensions of power as defined by Lukes (1974). He has made a fundamental statement on this topic and distinguishes between three dimensions in the execution of power. Actors in this context can be individuals, groups, organizations or political institutions, and they can act both intentionally and unintentionally. The one-dimensional form of power involves an instrumental attitude towards power where the practising of power involves actor A getting actor B to perform action x, even if he/she would prefer action y. One criterion for being able to talk about the execution of this sort of power is that it is observable. This means that there has to be a visible conflict between actors A and B, and that the action executed can be separated from the action superseded. This type of execution of power represents an operational form of power, where one actor has the power to control another actor's actions. We can also say that, in relation to the policy process model, this form of power represents the output side of the model; in other words, to what extent the political institution has the power to control how the solutions for actual problems are being carried out. The output side of the model can involve problem-solving in relation to the resolution, but can also involve symbolic problem-solving, escaping from the problem and unintended consequences. The execution of power can involve different asymmetric forms where one of the parts dominates the other, for instance through commandments, requests and teaching. But it can also involve negotiations between equal parts. Lukes (1974) calls this form of execution of power one-dimensional because it disregards other important forms of the execution of power.

In addition to one-dimensional power, two-dimensional power comes in the form of having the power to hinder the political system in making decisions that can solve the problem. In the policy process model, this power is expressed through having control over the decision-making activity, and, in other models, it can be called control over the throughput side of the policy process.

Three-dimensional power represents control over the political agenda. In relation to the policy-making model, this involves having control of the input side and the influence on, for instance, what people think and care about, and how strongly people argue their case. Execution of power of this dimension can prevent minorities from developing into majorities and, consequently, it can involve some anti-democratic patterns of action. On the other hand, the three-dimensional view of power allows people to mobilize and put their problems and solutions on the political agenda, eventually replace actors or set up new political institutions.

For the HEPRO project, one of the main goals was to put health high on the political and social agenda and to build a strong movement for public health at the local level. We argued that policy-making is a continual process, and it is not enough to put the values, needs and problems on the agenda; they have to be kept there, and the system must produce adequate outputs and outcomes over time. Therefore, there is a need for institutional changes that are able to implement the health policy.

Institutional capacity building in public health work

Labonte and Laverack (2001a,b) have delivered central work on *capacity building in health promotion*. In Labonte and Laverack (2001a: 112), they write that capacity in health promotion often is presumed to exist as an unproblematic resource that can be monitored and measured. However, more rigorous works describe capacity as social and organizational relations with dynamic qualities rather than static properties. Laverack has identified nine domains in a community capacity-building process, and, according to Labonte and Laverack (2001a: 130), these nine domains must combine the logic of health promotion top-down programmes with bottom-up mobilization and emancipation, in order to:

1   improve community participation;
2   develop local leadership;
3   build empowering organizational structures;
4   increase community members' problem assessment capacities;
5   enhance community members' ability to 'ask why';
6   improve community resource mobilization;
7   strengthen community links to other organizations and people;
8   create an equitable relationship with outside agents; and
9   increase community control over programme management.

Laverack and Labonte (2000: 257) argue that, in order to ensure *community capacity building* and *community empowerment*, it is best to see the process as an integrated *two-parallel structure*, with a programme track and an empowerment track that are linked during the progressive stages of the programme implementation process:

1   overall programme design
2   objective setting
3   strategy selection
4   strategy implementation
5   programme evaluation.

Their intention is to provide us with a planning framework for incorporating community empowerment into a top-down health promotion programme. We find this is a good description of some of the challenges of combining top-down and bottom-up implementation, but their framework seems to build on a linear form of planning, without discussing all the limitations such a linear process has when used on a continuous process such as public health work.

A more circular model is provided by Tones (1974) and Tones and Green (2004). They describe a systems checklist for health promotion. The model combines an education and cognitive affective behavioural change process, with an environment and supportive policy process. The model incorporates a lot of variables that we find relevant for a planning process, but the model may be too complex when used as an approach to health promotion planning.

In the field of regional planning science, Healey (1999) has presented a model of *institutional capacity building* in communities as a continuing process with different forms of capacity, which together add up to the institutional capacity:

- knowledge resources
- relations resources
- mobilization capability.

The knowledge and relations resources are, in this model, regarded as prerequisite for the *mobilization capacity*, and they all together form the strength of the institutional capacity. It is important for communities to have a strong, local institutional capacity in order to respond to external forces and internal evolution. However, the different forms of capacity will differ from community to community and from time to time. A weakness of this model is that institutional capacity seems, to a great extent, to be regarded as an endogenous process, and the model is unclear on how exogenous processes form the institutional capacity. The *'new public management'* (NPM) *reform* is one very important factor in the context of public health work that we have to take into consideration, and the political system model in Figure 1.2 can also be used to illustrate the outcome problem in the public sector caused by the NPM reform wave as the external force.

New public management and the outcome problem

The NPM reforms are in line with the general modernization of society and mean to seek objective knowledge that can enforce more cost-efficient production in the government structure. The NPM reforms brought new thinking and processes into the public sector, but many of them in the form of management borrowed from the private sector. In this process, the well-established terms *public sector* and *public administration* became discredited, and the private sector was put forward as an example to follow. The term 'public sector' became very much associated with an inefficient, rule-bound system, in contrast to the efficient private sector. The NPM reforms make marked competition an end in itself, and other ends such as democracy, participation and equality become more or less neglected. Thus, the NPM reforms make public and voluntary organizations become more like private sector organizations, with a dominance of instrumental rationality and internal focus.

Hence, the reforms focused on transforming the input-managed, rule-bound system into a more output- and even outcome-managed performance system. Management-by-objectives concepts and activity planning became central in the reforms. According to the Organization for Economic Co-operation and Development (OECD, 2003), this approach, with the emphasis on a formal system of specification of ends and measurement of output and outcome, failed decades ago, not only in the private sector, but also in the public sector in the command economies, because it could not address complex problems, and because there are limits on how much information human beings can (or do) take into account when they make decisions. In addition, there is no area of activity more complex than the policy domain of government, and it has, for a long time, been recognized that public service production is controlled more by values and culture than by rules, a situation that is likely to continue, despite progress in performance measurement and contracts. The OECD (2002) reports that, in many countries, the NPM reform has come to a standstill, and Norman (2006) reports from New Zealand, a country that was a *front runner* in the reform, that it now is accounting for outputs (efficiency), but is having a problem with measuring and managing the outcomes (effectiveness). The reform has increased '*silo thinking*', and public sector leaders are not kept accountable for the negative consequences of their sector-egoism. Increased sector thinking and acting, and a fragmentation of the national state seem to be common consequences of the NPM reforms across countries (Christensen and Lægreid, 2004).

It is commonly recognized that the public sector has a far more complex and dynamic value and goal structure than the private sector. There is now a growing awareness that something is missing between the existing public service culture and the public interests. There seems to be a lack of dedication among leaders to the fundamental values of public service, such as separated powers, democracy, transparency, accountability, equity and effectiveness. If these values are to guide the public sector actions, they must be embedded in the culture, and the public sector seems to have a very strong need for *institutional leadership*, that is leaders with the dedication and ability to put on the policy agenda the fundamental values of public services. Therefore, public health work becomes a leadership issue, and it becomes obvious that leaders must be involved in the process.

The spatial and cross-sectoral focus on public health

Public health work as a community empowerment process

Since the 1980s public administration leaders, health professionals, non-government agencies, government agencies, and so on have increasingly turned to empowerment and community participation as major strategies for alleviating poverty and social exclusion, and reducing health disparities. *Community development* has become a territory-based, multi-sector and multilevel approach that uses empowerment, planning and partnership to support and increase the community's ability to solve its own problems. In this new context, individuals and collectives have to take more responsibility for their own health and well-being. *Empowerment strategies*, participation, community development and other bottom-up approaches have become important in public health – this in contrast to the top-down strategies from the 1960s and 1970s.

In the *Declaration of Alma Ata*, the full participation of the community in the multidimensional work of health improvement became one of the pillars of public health work and the 'Health for all' movement (WHO, 1978). According to the *Jakarta declaration* (WHO, 1997), breaking down barriers between sectors and levels and creating partnerships were seen as essential for health promotion. *Partnership for health promotion* can be defined as voluntary agreements between two or more partners to work co-operatively towards a set of shared health outcomes, and these partnerships do work. They promote health across sectors, between professional and lay members, and between public, private and voluntary agencies at a collective level, as well as promoting individual health-related behaviour change (Gillies, 1998).

In the Ottawa Charter of health promotion, *health promotion* is defined as the process of enabling people to increase control over, and to improve, their health (WHO, 1986). In health promotion, partnerships for health and social development must be consolidated and expanded among different sectors at all community levels in order to create supportive environments for health. The main objective of this process is to empower people and communities, and to increase their control of the factors that create health. Community empowerment, planning and participation are seen, in the *Sundsvall statement on supportive environments for health*, as important factors in the health promotion approach, and the driving force for self-reliance and development (WHO, 1991).

In a report on the effectiveness of empowerment to improve health, the WHO quotes the World Bank, which defines empowerment as the process of increasing the capacity of individuals or groups to make choices, and to transform those choices into desired actions and outcomes; to build individual and collective assets; to improve the efficiency and fairness of the organizational and institutional contexts that govern the use of assets; and to achieve the expansion of assets and the capabilities of poor people to participate in, negotiate with, influence, control and hold accountable institutions that influence their lives (HEN, 2006: 17). From a review of the literature, the conclusions are that empowerment strategies are promising in their ability to produce both empowerment and health impacts, and that they are more likely to be successful if integrated within macro-economic and policy strategies aimed at creating greater equity (HEN, 2006: 14).

Empowerment in public health is an action-oriented concept, with a focus on the removal of formal or informal barriers, and on transforming power relations between communities and institutions and government. It is based on the assumption of community cultural assets that can be strengthened through dialogue and action (HEN, 2006: 18). The World Bank has identified four characteristics to ensure that participation is empowering (HEN, 2006: 9):

- people's access to information on public health issues;
- their inclusion in decision-making;
- local organizational capacity to make demands on institutions and governing structures; and
- accountability of institutions to the public.

Participation can make up the base of empowerment in public health, but is alone insufficient if the process does not build a capacity for further community actions. Participation is seen as a complex and interactive process that can grow or diminish based on the unfolding of power relations and the context of the project. Participation seems critical in reducing the dependency on health professionals and ensuring cultural and local sensitivity of programmes. Participation is not predictable in its outcomes and happens with or without professionals. Therefore, professionals' roles in the community development process must shift from dominant to supportive or facilitative (HEN, 2006: 8).

In public health work, *community empowerment interventions* are regarded as complex, dynamic and comprehensive. This is a multilevel and multi-sector approach involving individuals, communities, states, and so on, and public, private and voluntary sectors in governance structures and processes. Case studies seem to show that integrated programmes, with synergy between anti-poverty strategies, NGO and government collaboration and community participation, are probably most effective in improving health and development outcomes (HEN, 2006: 15).

Hyung Hur (2006) discusses the term 'empowerment' from theoretical perspectives. John Friedmann's work on empowerment is one of the theoretical perspectives that are included in that discussion. Friedmann (1992) has an in-depth discussion of empowerment from the perspective of modernization of the society where the *instrumental, top-down policy* dominates the *communicative, bottom-up policy*. His solution is a better balance between instrumental and communicative rationality, a solution that gets support from Jürgen Habermas (1984; 1987; 1995).

Prilleltensky (2005) discusses the promotion of well-being and concludes that reactive, individual, alienating and deficit-based approaches that foster patienthood instead of health, citizenship and democracy have dominated the field of health services for decades, and that it is time to shift paradigms and give strength-based, preventive, empowering and community-oriented approaches a chance to promote personal, relational and collective well-being.

According to Huang and Wang (2005: 13), public health services (such as health education and primary care) in community-based settings traditionally focus on the deficiencies of individuals, treatment of sick individuals and problem-solving by outside experts. These emphases undermine the clients' sense of capacity and self-worth, decrease their involvement in decision-making about health, limit use of resources from the community and weaken community ties. Now, primary health care, health promotion and community development have been integrated into community health practice. All three approaches to health care involve strengthening community competence and creating community change (Huang and Wang, 2005: 15).

In community development, health promotion is more concerned with community empowerment than changes in particular disease risks and un-healthy lifestyles. However, according to Laverack and Labonte (2000: 261), the empowerment discourse of health promoters, legitimized by the *Ottawa Charter for Health Promotion* (WHO, 1986), has created a major tension in health promotion today. Many health promoters continue to exert power over the community through top-down programmes, while at the same time inviting people into emancipatory, bottom-up processes, without having a clear understanding of how community empowerment can be accommodated within health promotion programmes. Two seemingly different health promotion discourses coexist and have evolved into two distinct and somewhat exclusive approaches that are problematic to combine in practice (Laverack and Labonte, 2000: 256):

1 The *conventional discourse* emphasizes top-down disease prevention through lifestyle management and vector control.
2 The *communicative discourse* emphasizes social justice through bottom-up community empowerment, advocacy and partnership.

These are two discourses that also exist in planning research (see, among others, Sager (1990) for a fundamental discussion) and the conclusion and the great challenge is how to combine the top-down and bottom-up approaches. In accordance with that conclusion, we understand community-oriented public health work, such as the HEPRO project, as a combination of top-down and bottom-up policy-making, and as a broad social learning and mobilization activity that is supposed to enhance the individual and collective capacity in local and regional communities to take care of public health (see Figure 1.3).

In the HEPRO project, we argued for using the term empowerment in line with Friedmann (1992). Empowerment thus implies a gathering of power in a dynamic way, over a period of time, in a combination of external support and internal mobilization. Empowerment implies an increase in consciousness, but it implies more than a change of power in which there

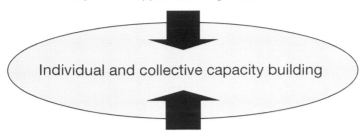

Figure 1.3 Empowerment as capacity building

is a destruction of previous structures and values. People become empowered when they move up the spiral to a higher level of self-understanding. Or, to put it very simply, the best everyday definition of empowerment is very simple – 'helping people to help themselves' or 'leading people to learn to lead themselves'.

The HEPRO project is what is often called a *programme* in the public health literature. In a categorization of programmes by level of community involvement created by Tones and Green (2004: 261), the HEPRO project can be characterized as a type 1 programme, with high community involvement and with a major goal to empower people and improve the socio-economic conditions. But we know from our research on regional development programmes that, in spite of the good intentions, the programme was in danger of ending up as a type 5 programme in the referred category of programmes, a programme type delivering preventive services directly to clients and with a limited outreach.

The situation in the public health work that we have described is quite similar to the recent situation in regional planning and development work. The operating principles of EU regional policy involve greater delegation to the regions and mobilization of organizations to work in partnerships. These principles have led to the establishment of regional structures for planning and implementation of regional policies. Uyarra (2007: 256) concludes, in her critical discussion on regional innovation policies, that there is a need to better investigate the formulation and implementation of innovation policies in a multilevel, multi-actor context, and a need to understand better the diversity of the regional context.

Sectoral and spatial planning – a two-parallel system

The regional planning systems in the Nordic countries can illustrate a number of recent changes that point towards increased similarities with other

European planning systems, and the systems can illustrate how the two discourses coexist also in regional planning. The most obvious change is the emergence of a regional level, a trend that is definitely related to European spatial development policies (Böhme, 2002). In addition, Böhme points to another trend that has become evident: the increasing cross-sectoral perspective. It may be too early to talk about a trend towards overcoming the strong sector orientation of Nordic spatial policy, but there are at least initial signs of approaches to a more integrated spatial planning.

The term *regional planning* is used to cover *spatial regional planning* and *sectoral regional planning* (R. Amdam, 2004). Spatial planning focuses on the region as a society, and sectoral planning focuses on planning in organizations in the society (municipalities, counties, etc.). We find this use of the terms to be in accordance with a common understanding of spatial planning:

> Spatial planning refers to the methods used largely by the public sector to influence the future distribution of activities in space. It is undertaken with the aims of creating a more rational territorial organization of land uses and the linkages between them, to balance demands for development with the need to protect the environment, and to achieve social and economic objectives. Spatial planning embraces measures to co-ordinate the spatial impacts of other sectoral policies, to achieve a more even distribution of economic development between regions than would otherwise be created by market forces, and to regulate the conversion of land and property uses.
>
> (European Community, 1997: 24)

The European Spatial Development Perspective (ESDP) was adopted in May 1999 in Potsdam by the informal Council of EU Ministers responsible for spatial planning, and the shaping of the perspective has been a fragile and uncertain process. The ESDP creates a common vocabulary of symbols and visions in the discourse of European spatial development, and the perspective has a triangle of objectives linking the following fundamental goals of European policy (European Community, 1999: 10):

- economic and social cohesion;
- conservation of natural resources and cultural heritage; and
- more balanced competitiveness of the European territory.

These objectives are further developed in spatial development guidelines and specified in a number of policy aims and options (European Community, 1999: 11). One of the guidelines is the development of a polycentric and balanced urban system and strengthening of the partnership between urban and rural areas. This involves overcoming the outdated dualism between city and countryside. In order to understand these perspectives and guidelines, we have to remember that the long-term spatial development trends in the EU are, above all, influenced by three processes:

- the progressive economic integration and related increased co-operation between the member states;
- the growing importance of local and regional communities and their role in spatial development; and
- the enlargement of the EU and the development of closer relations with its neighbours.

The translation of the objectives and options into concrete political action will take place gradually. The ESDP will, therefore, periodically be subject to review. However, we have to remember that EU polity is a complex, multilevel institutional configuration that cannot be adequately represented by the theoretical models that are generally used in international relations and comparative policies (Scharpf, 2001: 20). The models that exist will have specific implications for how we regard the institutional capacity and legitimacy of the European governing functions. The separation of political power between the different levels will nevertheless be an important issue in spatial planning and development. The integrated policy concept of ESDP, as mentioned above, requires new ways of co-operation between levels and new ways of handling sectoral and spatial conflicts. The application of the policy options is based on the principle of subsidiarity and, according to the ESDP's principles, the implementation will be on a voluntary basis. There is thus a need for close co-operation among the authorities responsible for sectoral policies; and between those responsible for spatial development at each respective level (horizontal co-operation); and between actors at the Community level and the transnational, regional and local levels (vertical co-operation).

The European Spatial Planning Observation Network (ESPON) has been set up with the purpose of providing an analytical base for the ESDP agenda and has produced significant data. Meanwhile, however, the work on establishing a constitution for Europe has identified territorial cohesion as an objective for the EU, and the ESDP agenda has been modified under the flag of *territorial cohesion* (Faludi, 2006).

Regardless, from our point of view, there are several problems in the planning system deriving from the ESDP and territorial cohesion policy. First, we have the *horizontal co-ordination problem*, when the regional policy-making and implementing are expanded from the public sector to include the voluntary and private sectors in networks and partnerships. Then, we have the *vertical co-ordination problem*, with the extremely difficult balance between top-down and bottom-up policies in the multilevel power structure of the EU. Last, we have the problem with creating processes and institutions with enough acceptance, power and legitimacy to co-ordinate vertically and horizontally. This can be called the *policy instrument problem.*

Public health work and regional planning and development do, in this field, face the same challenges in modern societies. Regional territorial and horizontal power seems to be weak compared with sectoral and vertical power, and it can be argued that the situation in general is a consequence of the *modernization* process in our societies (Giddens, 1997; Habermas, 1984; 1987; 1995). In this process, instrumental rationality and top-down policy seem to dominate communicative rationality and bottom-up policy. In order to understand these challenges fully, we have to clarify the terms 'instrumental rationality' and 'communicative rationality'.

Modernization and instrumental versus communicative rationality

Instrumental rationality tells us how to combine the means to achieve given ends, and it is appropriate for goal-oriented behaviour within a means–end structured problem area. Planning based on instrumental rationality can lead to bigger local and regional dependency on external institutions and forces. According to Stöhr (1990), it can also weaken local communities' capability to learn and to handle challenges. Dryzek (1990) blames instrumental rationality for many of the crises in the world and argues that the cure is communicative rationality and discursive democracy with participatory democracy, communicative action and practical reasoning. The term *communicative rationality* comes from Habermas (1984; 1987), who argues that communicative rationality is a property of inter-subjective discourses, not individual maximization, and it can pertain to the generation of normative judgements and action principles rather than just to the selection of means to an end. Communicative rationality is rooted in the inter-action of social life and is oriented towards inter-subjective understanding, the co-ordination of actions through discussion, and the socialization of members of the community. However, communicative rationality cannot totally replace instrumental rationality; it can only restrict the latter to a subordinate domain (Habermas, 1995).

Instrumental rationality points towards the gains that society can achieve through economy and science and has formed the foundation for under-standing modernizing as an expression of progress, and that progress is associated with better efficiency and rationalization. If we use instrumental rationality as a foundation for reforms in the 'modern state', the state will become a more efficient instrument to produce output and outcome. However, many scientists argue that this is not enough to legitimate the modern state. In addition, we have to raise the question of to what extent the state has become more democratic, just and humane. Eriksen (1993) substantiates this by asking if there is enough done to ensure that every group and its needs, interests and demands for respect are being looked after. Eriksen also asks if public sector activities are in accordance with valid moral and standard court justice. He finds great shortages in today's presumption of modernizing, and he argues strongly for the usage of other forms of rationality, especially communicative rationality.

Friedmann (1992) states that modern society suffers under instrumental rationality and the neglect of communicative rationality and collective processes. He argues that the solution to the problem is to mobilize territorial power to meet sectoral power in a political process. In a local and regional policy context and in public health work, this means that the bottom-up, mainly communicative, power can equalize with the top-down, mainly instrumental, power and thus contribute to the building of adequate regional development institutions.

From this perspective, it becomes logical to empower local and regional communities to oppose the dominant vertical, mainly instrumental, power structure (Friedmann and Weaver, 1979). This involves a strengthening of the *horizontal power structure* through the activation of civil society and elected representatives, and through local embedding of private businesses. In this way, horizontal political power can be organized to supplement and oppose the sector-dominated and *vertical power structure*. Many researchers agree upon this point of view and see the local community, with a strong civil society and a strong democratic process, as the main key to empower local and regional communities (see, among others, Bennett and McCoshan (1993), Forester (1993), Putnam (1993) and Storper (1997)).

Instrumental rationality is the logic of *the traditional linear model of planning*. In the linear model, the focus is on relating means (how to do something) to ends (what could be achieved), in logical and systematic ways. Scientific knowledge will provide an objective basis for identifying present problems and predicting future possibilities (see Figure 1.4).

A prerequisite for this planning is, among other things, that, at the moment of decision, there is full awareness of the present situation and clear and unambiguous objectives for the future, so that it is possible to choose which alternative offers the best course of action (Simon, 1965).

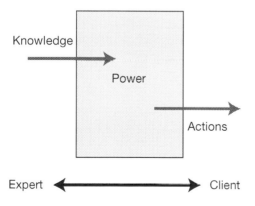

Figure 1.4 Positivist epistemology and instrumental planning

Instrumental rationality and planning are strongly connected with the positivists' theory of knowledge. The presumption here is that objective knowledge can be gained through a scientific, hypothetical-deductive process. The controlled experiment stands as the methodical ideal. The founding doctrine for positivism is to clear the world of religion and mysticism, and to achieve control of society through knowledge and technique. The only true views of the world are those that are based on empirical observations. Assertions that are not testable in an analytical or empirical way shall be disregarded entirely. This positivist science ideal generates an interest in research aimed at unveiling connections between cause and effect, and establishing 'laws of societies'.

Instrumental rationality has a strong position in public health work and is decisive when society needs evidence-based knowledge to intervene in processes in order to prevent people from suffering illness and injury. Forbidding people to smoke in public places is a very good example of successful, evidence-based intervention and health prevention.

However, Friedmann (1978) states that *the positivist epistemology* is too dominant in our time. He writes that this epistemology has three levels or worlds: practice, technology and science (World 1, World 2 and World 3). Real science and objective knowledge can be found in World 3. World 2 uses this knowledge to develop techniques, and World 1 is the world where the techniques are practised. This epistemology is based on the definition of objective knowledge. This means that it is possible to come up with knowledge that is independent of any knowing subject.

Schön (1983) claims that this epistemology has led to practice as an instrumental professional activity, where the process of solving problems is made rigorous by the use of science, theory and technique. The owners of the scientific knowledge have formed professions based on, among others, the following characteristics: basic knowledge, used science and action competence. Some of these actors have, through use of the positivist science ideal, made systemized bases of knowledge with four important capabilities. The knowledge is *specialized*, *stabilized*, *standardized* and *scientific*. These actors have made what Schön calls '*over-professions*' based on codified knowledge (medical doctors, engineers, etc.). Some of the other actors work in what can be called '*under-professions*'. We will say that typical examples of these 'under-professions' are planners, public health and social workers, and any others who base their knowledge on participation in social interaction. These professions are not capable of forming a basis for systematic scientific knowledge, because the same actions will give different results in different contexts. The competence of action is weakened this way, because the coherence between knowledge and actions is complex and labile, and much of the adequate knowledge is tacit, and personally and locally embedded.

Schön (1983) asks us eagerly to admit the weaknesses of instrumental rationality and rather seek for an epistemology that is based upon practice in creativity and intuitiveness similar to those that the practitioner uses when facing unique situations with uncertainty, conflict and instability. Schön introduces and uses the word *reflective practitioner* and writes that, when we reflect during actions, we ourselves become researchers in a practical context. We think of what we can do while we do it. We do not depend upon theories or techniques; we make theory out of cases. This method of rationality is suitable for handling uncertainty, because it does not separate ends and means, knowledge and actions, planning and implementation from each other. These are developed interactively. After a while, we will have both a *codified* and a *tacit knowledge* that we base our actions upon. However, the tacit knowledge can be a weakness with the reflective practitioner. Specialists, for instance, have a great deal of uncodified, tacit knowledge based on earlier experiences. Thus, they can be regarded as boring, exhausted and over-educated, and they can also have been dragged into patterns of action with mistakes they cannot correct, and therefore become inattentive to situations not fitting into their established patterns of action. The reflective practitioner must therefore involve him- or herself with communicative situations where these irrational actions can be revealed and corrected.

Schön (1983) suggests that instrumental rationality is a process for problem-solving, but not for problem-formulating. He claims this by saying that instrumental models of action do not catch the real world. The model cannot handle uncertainty in the forms of non-stability and complexity, and it is not capable of handling conflicting needs, interests and values. Schön adds that instrumental rationality is not the only point of view existing: there are other competing forms of rationality.

Schön (1986) does not refer to Friedmann's work, but the intention of Friedmann (1978) was to make an alternative epistemology for use in social contexts as a substitute for the epistemology occupied with objective knowledge based on the positivist science ideal. Friedmann (1978; 1987; 1992) rejects the positivist science ideal and, thus, also the deductive research design's approach to obtain objective knowledge through verifying and falsifying hypotheses. Friedmann put forward the *epistemology of social practice* as an alternative to positivist epistemology. Friedmann writes that this epistemology can be traced back to Aristotle, because social practice refers to moral actions in public spheres, and because actions are based on norms regarding how we are supposed to live alongside each other. Friedmann's epistemological model has only one 'world' and one living theory that places the facts inside the world. In this model, learning is linked to events via social actions and the result of those actions. The adequacy of the theory of reality and/or the political strategy is therefore dependent on the results of action and the extent to which these results satisfy the given social values.

Friedmann argues for constant critical evaluation and successive revision of the components in the model. The social practice epistemology is a model for *social learning*, where the learning happens with interaction between radical practice and critical reflection (see the model in Figure 1.5). The model shows that social practice grows through continuous critical evaluation and successive revision of the components in the model as they malfunction. The model results in *personal growth* owing to the fact that the participants tie together knowledge and actions when they alternate between critical acknowledging and new practice. Friedmann suggests further that, even if the epistemology regarding social practice exceeds the epistemology dealing with objective knowledge, it is far from a substitute.

Communicative planning is rooted in the epistemology of social practice and is not carried out by experts for the objective of the plan, but in face-to-face dialogue between those involved and interested. Personal growth and joint action are the key elements in this planning. Communicative (or deliberative) planning is based on the assumption that better decisions are reached if they emerge out of a dialogue between those concerned. Rather than a technocratic process carried out by planners, planning is regarded as an interactive, communicative process. The planning process will transform knowledge into action through an uninterrupted sequence of relationships between people. The planning is not divorced from other social action in which the aim is to gain control over social processes that affect one's welfare. Communicative planning emphasizes a broad, grass-roots mobilization to gain the strength to take greater responsibility for one's development and to influence the conditions under which one is working. Knowledge and action can be linked through critical understanding and radical practice, and the planning process is a far-reaching learning process in which everyone can participate. Without a vision, there is no radical practice; without radical practice, no formation of a theory; without a theory, no strategy; and without a strategy, no action. These relationships can be illustrated as a learning spiral (see Figure 1.5).

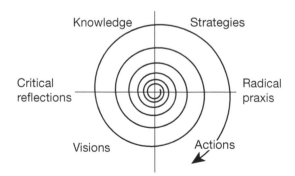

Figure 1.5 Social practice epistemology and communicative planning
Source: After Friedmann (1978: 87)

Friedmann points out the following advantages of this model (1978: 87):

- Knowledge and actions can be tied to a model for democratic processes.
- Knowledge grows from conflicting incidents and thus has a political dimension.
- Anyone who wants to can participate, and there exists no monopoly, nor distinguished elite.
- The separation between objective and subjective knowledge disappears, and abstract and concrete knowledge are combined in a single process of learning and practising.
- Normative contributions will not be smuggled in, but will openly be presented for criticism.
- The model can be used in formulations of theories. What is learned in one situation can be abstract knowledge in another.

Friedmann gets support for his ideas about the reflective practitioner from, among others, Bolan (1980), who writes about the *practitioner as theorist*. He also starts by saying that the difference between theory and practice, knowledge and actions is bigger than ever. He asserts further that, if we make planning a professional and instrumental problem-solver, one effect could be that citizens would become less self-sufficient and that they would come into a structural relationship of dependency towards professional helpers. This effect could eventually become stronger, making the distance between knowledge and actions even greater. He maintains that every incident is special, and the most meaningful theories are those that are constructed in the minds of the practitioners and that have been tried out in practice. He says that professional practice is guided by knowledge, and that knowledge is formed by practice. However, norms, interests and values control actions; thus, the planner should not only be regarded as an instrumental planner, but also as a politician representing norms, interests and values.

Friedmann (1992) has written an important contribution on empowerment. He joins the criticism of the modernization of society and adds that a relative strengthening is taking place of the instrumental logic that now permeates private enterprises and public sector administration. He believes that this has a negative effect on the communicative common sense, which, in the main, is kept alive in democratic governing bodies and in civil society. Developing this thesis still further, he claims that the modernization has led to an increased emphasis on instrumental rationality and the promoting of self-interest, with less emphasis being placed on a fellowship that forms morals and on collective interests. Friedmann believes the key to further development now is to strengthen the relations between the social power in civil society and the political power in democratically elected governing bodies.

Furthermore, he maintains that politics should lead to the formation of a moral fellowship and that political activity cannot, therefore, be reduced to the economic calculation of utilitarian value and sociological determinism. However, Friedmann himself is aware that the strengthening of relations between the civil society and the people's democratically elected representatives often meets strong opposition from the establishment. Seen in relation to planning, this will involve strengthening planning's territorial dimension at the expense of the sector dimension. To put it another way, cross-sector co-ordination can only be achieved by creating a territorial counterbalance to the vertical and sector-based governance structure.

System and life world and the political will-forming process

Habermas (1984; 1987) joins the general critics of modern society. He claims that the positivist cognitive theory increases the distance between theory and practice, and that the formation of policy in modern society is fragmented and instrumental. Habermas uses the terms 'system' and 'life world' to describe this development. By *system*, he means economic and political-administrative activity based on the steering media money and power, and demands for results aiming at the goals of functional ability and efficiency. This system is characterized by the maximization of individual benefit and instrumental rationality, and it is capable of creating systemic integration. In the *life world*, co-ordinated action builds on consensus created on the basis of ideal conversations. The focus is on the participants, and they are involved in communicative relations with each other. This results in a *social integration*, as opposed to *systemic integration*, and builds on an unspoken, common evaluation of the situation, common goals and values, and so on. The life world is tied to civil society and open, free, democratic processes.

Habermas claims that the system *colonizes* the life world, and that instrumental rationality thus displaces communicative rationality. As a counterweight to this development, he wants to strengthen the public sphere in society. By *public sphere*, he means the social room created by actors acting communicatively. Thus, the public sphere does not become a separate institution or organization to which we can relate by studying structure, processes, norms, rules, etc. The public sphere is rather a network of communication and a process of interaction that assist in putting issues on the political agenda and ensure that solutions are passed and implemented, but also that the consequences are debated and evaluated. It is in the public sphere that moral judgements of what is fair, right, democratic, and so on will be expressed most clearly. We can thus claim that the public sphere represents the centre of democracy (Eriksen, 1994: 16), but it has to be added that the public sphere can be abused and manipulated, but it cannot be subjected to open pressure without the actors having to show themselves and so weaken the force of their arguments.

Through his theory of communicative action, Habermas tries to develop concepts for understanding how norms and solidarity are created communally. Behind this is an assumption that consensus is possible, and that the actors want to achieve a common will. Many critics of such consensus building claim that this can be possible and desirable only in small groups. In his book *Between facts and norms*, Habermas returns to the problems he set out discussing earlier, that is, the necessary conditions for rational communication on the problems of society, and the meaning of democracy (Habermas, 1995). The perspective here is that, with the construction of the democratic, constitutional state in a modern society, institutional arrangements for legitimizing this constitutional state have arisen. The line of reasoning is that no external authorities exist that guarantee the legitimacy of the democratic constitutional state. It has to secure its legitimacy on its own through *free processes of public will formation*. However, the public opinion-making process has little chance of being directly transformed into political action. The communicative power from the free opinion-making process in the political public sphere is through the passage of laws and regulations transformed into administrative power in the shape of state power to organize, sanction and implement. This means that it is not the individual morality of the actors that decides the ability to act collectively and in solidarity, but rather the procedures for democratic will formation and collective decision-making, which are institutionalized in modern societies. In this way, Habermas arrives at the normative point of view that a society should vitalize the connection between civil society and the political system through institutional reforms.

Habermas's *theory of communicative action* tries to develop an extended universalistic concept of rationality that not only covers instrumental rationality, but also communicative rationality (Habermas, 1984; 1987; 1995). This is probably one reason why his theory is strongly criticized, but also eagerly embraced by many. A recurring line of argument in his works is based on the concepts of *speech act* and communicative rationality. He proceeds from the basis that speech is an act. Whoever expresses him- or herself verbally will, through this speech act, communicate a connection to an objective world of existing facts and circumstances, to a subjective world of personal experiences and emotions, and to a social world of accepted and valid norms. The listeners can evaluate how the statement relates to *communicative validity claims*, that is, that a speech act must be *true*, *sincere*, *right* and *comprehensible*.

The listeners have the option to contradict what is said by means of a new speech act, and the actors will thus become involved in a process with a mutual duty to give arguments for one's statements and with rules of procedure defined by the validity claims. To argue against these claims will mean involving oneself in contradictions. The actors thus do not relate their statements directly to existing self-interests or norms, but instead relate the statement to the possibility that the validity claims will be countered by others. In this way, instrumental rationality, with its focus on facts and truth, meets with communicative rationality, with its focus on sincerity, legitimacy and comprehensibility. Facts and truth are almost always dependent on paradigmatic values, morals and views, and that is why communicative rationality has to be made superior to instrumental rationality (Dryzek, 1990; Friedmann, 1992; Habermas, 1995).

Communicative rationality emphasizes the meaningful and action-co-ordinating potential of the speech acts themselves. Through discourse, the conversation partners may arrive at common understandings of adequate actions, by which they feel bound. Communicative rationality can contribute to building moral-forming communities, and to integrating individual and collective values, interests and needs, but such a product assumes that the discourse can be understood as an ideal conversation that, in addition to the duty to argue, also builds on parity of power and public sphere.

From the work of Habermas (1984; 1987; 1995), one can draw the conditions for the *undistorted discourse*. All individuals who can speak and act are to be free to participate, free to question any proposal, free to make any proposal, and free to express their attitudes, desires and needs. No speaker is to be hindered by force, either from inside or outside the discourse, from making use of these conditions.

Parity of power is important for the conversation to become a dialogue where the force of argument in the relationship between the actors decides the outcome of the conversation, not the power of one participant to force his or her views and norms on others. Furthermore, the ideal conversation presupposes a public sphere, so that the *duty to argue* applies even outside this particular group of persons in this particular discourse. This means that none of the actors is to execute any power in the discourse that makes any other actor become structurally subordinate, and that the weightiest argument ideally should be given the most weight in the process of forming consensus. The demand for reason, together with the demand for publicity, forces the participants to defend their statements towards citizens who are not taking part in the discourses.

In this political will-forming and legitimating model, Habermas talks about different *discourses* with their respective rationalities, which together form a political legitimating process (see Figure 1.6). Habermas understands the political process as a will-formation process starting with *pragmatic* discourses that further lead to *ethical* discourses and to *moral* discourses, depending on the kinds of conflict present. These discourses can lead to *juridical* discourses, which are oriented towards the consistency of laws and regulations. *Procedure-regulated negotiation* can be an alternative to discourses if these do not produce sufficient consensus (Eriksen, 1994).

We regard legitimacy, discourses, participation, action and learning as key issues in planning, and planning as an institution-building process. The planning process will serve to build up social, institutional and political capacity, which can become a new local and regional institutional resource and political power. Healey (1997: 314) calls this a *soft infrastructure*, but, without attention to the *hard infrastructure* represented by the formal policy

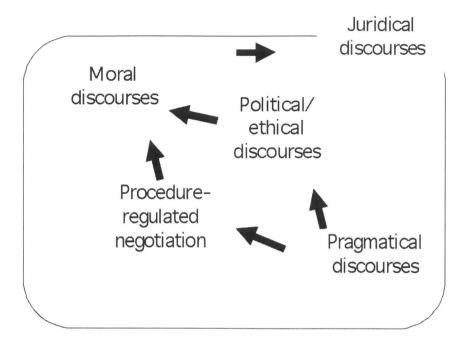

Figure 1.6 Discourses in a will-forming and political legitimating process
Source: After Habermas (1992: 207)

structure, it will be difficult to change current policy. These formal systems are often seen as immovable constraints that are simply just 'there'. However, these constraints are never fixed; they are socially constructed and they can be reconstructed through dialogue, mobilization and learning, and by the use of social, political and administrative power.

Scambler (2001a) has edited a book about Habermas, critical theory and health, which we value as a major contribution to the understanding of the fundamental challenges in public health work. In the introductory chapter of the book, Scambler writes an overview of Habermas's voluminous production, and he discusses central terms in Habermas's contribution to the development of critical theory. The overview consists of terms such as system, life world, public sphere, rationality, legitimation crises and, of course, the theory of communicative action, and Scambler tries to relate these terms to public health work (Scambler, 2001b). However, ideal conversations and policy legitimating processes are not an easy way to create a collective will (Jacobsson, 1997). In societies and communities that are based on democratic values, communicative action is the main approach to legitimating politics, laws and plans. Democracy and publicity are the best guarantees against illegitimate execution of power.

Basic assumptions and challenges

According to the WHO (1986), we define public health work as the creation and implementation of a healthy public policy for all. In this work, the public sector has limited resources, and people are now expected to take more responsibility for their own health; empowerment is put forward as an important approach in order to increase the individual and collective capacity to act. However, empowerment is a contested term, and empowerment is often understood as a mainly bottom-up process. We argue that this is too narrow an interpretation of the term.

In Western countries' political power structure, regional territorial and horizontal power is weak compared with sectoral and vertical power. It can be argued that the situation in general is a consequence of the modernization process in our societies (see Giddens, 1997). In this process, instrumental rationality and top-down policy seem to dominate over communicative rationality and bottom-up policy. Modern societies suffer under instrumental rationalities and the neglect of communicative rationalities and collective processes. Friedmann (1992) and Habermas (1995), for example, argue that the solution to the problem is to mobilize territorial power to meet sectoral power in a political process.

Our basic assumption is that a policy process and an empowerment process consist of a combination of top-down and bottom-up processes, and, in addition, we regard public health work as a combination of *prevention of ill health* and *promotion of good health*. We have delivered philosophical, theoretical and practical arguments for this assumption. The arguments can be summarized as follows: health prevention needs evidence-based knowledge about the relations between causes and effects in order to legitimize intervention, such as banning smoking in public places, and prevention is, in theory and practice, based on instrumental rationality. In health promotion, the causality between cause and effect is unclear and is often constructed in the social practice, and promotion is, to a large extent, based on communicative rationality. However, it is to simplify too much to say that prevention is an evidence-based, instrumental, top-down and sectorized activity, and that promotion is a communicative, bottom-up practice with broad participation in community development. From the discussion of the modernization process, we know that communicative and instrumental rationalities are interdependent, more like yin and yang, and that the major challenge is to combine them.

We argued that the HEPRO project needed to understand empowerment as a balanced combination of soft and hard infrastructure, of top-down and bottom-up policies, and of instrumental and communicative rationalities. The implication of this understanding is that, when the project is ended, the communities will have a better capacity to lead themselves, focus their challenges, organize themselves and implement actions, and learn from their experiences. In order to achieve this situation, it can be fruitful, as the

HEPRO project did, to regard the project as cross-sectoral and cross-level policy-making, and as an institution-building process supported by a circular planning approach. However, there is no single answer on how to balance the top-down and bottom-up policies, but the combination needs to be sorted out in the actual situation and context. One of the major changes in the context of regional development and public health work now is what can be called the *governance turn*, which we will discuss in the next chapter.

2 The governance turn in regional planning and public health

In the first chapter, we wrote that health promotion is now understood as empowerment, takes the form of community development and makes partnerships between the public, private and voluntary sectors' important tools in the development process. This can be interpreted as an attempt by the public sector to involve other sectors in the health promotion work, to share the responsibility for people's health with the other sectors, and to stimulate people to take more responsibility for their own health. This is similar to a process known from regional development and is often called the 'governance turn' in regional policies. In this chapter, our intention is to explore to what extent experiences from regional planning and development work can be transferred to public health work and become relevant knowledge for problem-solving there. In order to address this question, we first of all discuss the terms 'government' and 'governance'. Then, we summarize some of the findings from research done on implementing governance in public health, and we compare these findings with experiences from regional planning and development.

Introduction

In the EU, the operating principles of the regional policy involve greater delegation of responsibility to the regions and partnerships between sector, and between levels of government. The old paradigm of state intervention and distributed growth has been replaced with the paradigm based on endogenous growth and regions as strategic actors. Under this new regime, the regions can increase their competitive potential if they are able to produce their own institutional capacity for economic governance (Amin, 1999).

According to the United Nations (2009: 6), the most commonly recognized change in planning has been the expansion of the political system from 'government' to 'governance', which represents a response to the growing complexity of governing in a globalizing and multilevel context, as well as the involvement of a range of non-state actors in the process of governing. The concept of governance has been promoted along with decentralization and democratization, driven largely by multilateral institutions such as the

World Bank and International Monetary Fund. The principal ideas were privatization, deregulation and decentralization.

In political theory, the term *government* refers to the formal institutions of the state and their monopoly of legitimate coercive power. Government is the formal institutional structure and location of authoritative decision-making in the modern state, such as ministries, agencies, municipalities and counties. The concept of *governance*, in contrast, is wider and directs attention to the distribution of power, both internal and external to the state. Governance is about governmental and non-governmental organizations (NGOs) working together in a new planning and implementing structure based on partnership between the public, private and voluntary sectors, and between national, regional and local levels. The focus is on the interdependence of governmental and non-governmental forces in meeting economic and social challenges (Stoker, 1997: 10). Governance is always an interactive process, because no single actor, public or private, has the knowledge and resource capacity to tackle problems unilaterally. The governance concept points to the creation of new structures that are a result of the interaction of different actors. Recognizing the power dependence in collective actions implies accepting that intentions do not always match outcomes (Stoker, 1998: 22).

However, the term 'governance' is understood in two different ways: in a descriptive sense, it refers to the proliferation of institutions, agencies, interests and regulatory systems. In a normative sense, it refers to an alternative model for managing collective affairs. It is seen as horizontal self-organization among mutually interdependent actors, of which government is only one and with only imperfect control. This new form of governance has become necessary because of the restructuring of the state and has been reflected in a number of ways, such as (United Nations, 2009: 73):

- a relative decline in the role of formal government in the management of social and economic relationships;
- the involvement of non-governmental actors in a range of state functions at a variety of spatial levels;
- a change from hierarchical forms of government structures to more flexible forms of partnership and networking;
- a shift from provision by formal government structures to sharing of responsibilities and service provision between the state and civil society; and
- the devolution and decentralization of formal governmental responsibility to regional and local governments.

In regional planning and development, there has been an obvious swing from government to governance. As far as we can see, the same process is going on in public health work (Haines *et al.*, 2004; Vega and Irwin, 2004). The intention is seemingly to supplement the traditional government structure in public health with a governance structure. However, from regional policy research, we know that this change from government to governance is not without problems and challenges. Swyngedouw (2005) discusses the *Janus face* of governance and concludes that, instead of enhanced democracy, the extension of 'holder' participation and improved transparency, governance can become elite technocracy and power-based interest intermediation, and can face considerable internal and external problems with respect to accountability and legitimacy.

The governance turn

In Western democracies' regional policy-making and planning, a regional governance structure has been added to the regional government structure, and this so-called shift of regime started in the 1970s. It was then that the dominant accumulation regime, with its emphasis on large-scale enterprises and mass production, was hit by economic stagnation and staff reductions in large companies. Focus then was given to a more flexible accumulation regime, with great emphasis on innovation and growth in employment in small and medium-sized companies in clusters (Stöhr, 1990).

The shift of regime has had consequences for our perspective on governing, planning, policy-making, organization, and so on (Bukve and Amdam, 2004a; 2004b). The discussion of the governance turn in public health and regional development in this chapter is structured around five propositions, as identified by Stoker (1998) in his paper on governance. The aim is to present a number of aspects of governance and to discuss important challenges public health work is facing when it turns from government to governance. The five positions are (Stoker, 1998: 18):

1   Governance refers to a set of institutions and actors that are drawn from, but also beyond, government.
2   Governance identifies the blurring of boundaries and responsibilities for tackling social and economic issues.
3   Governance identifies the power dependence involved in the relationship between institutions involved in collective action.
4   Governance is about autonomous, self-governing networks of actors.
5   Governance recognizes the capacity to get things done that does not rest on the power of government to command and use its authority. It sees government as able to use new tools and techniques to steer and guide.

Governance refers to a set of institutions and actors that are drawn from, but also beyond, government

In regional policy, the term governance is used in a variety of ways, but there is baseline agreement that governance refers to the development of governing styles in which boundaries between and within the public sector have become blurred. The concept of governance has gained widespread currency across many of the social sciences, and many disciplines have struggled to analyse the broad set of changes in the relationship between state, market and civil society – the conceptual trinity that has tended to dominate mainstream analysis of modern societies.

In the concept of governance, actors and institutions attempt to establish a capacity to act by blending their resources, skills and purposes into a viable and sustainable partnership. This co-ordination process has been characterized, rather neatly, as 'managing a nobody-in-charge world' (Stoker, 1997). Some authors warn that the growing obsession with governance mechanisms as a solution to *market failure* or *state failure* should not lead us to neglect the possibility of *governance failure*. We must avoid seeing governance as necessarily being a more efficient solution to problems of economic or political co-ordination than markets or states. We must ask critical questions about those institutions and networks that emerge in their place (Jessop, 1997). Failures of leadership, differences in time scale and horizons among key partners, and the depth of social conflicts can all provide the seed for governance failures (Stoker, 1998: 24).

The NPM reforms have been a significant driving force in the transformation of public sector from government to governance. The label 'new public management' was first used by Hood (1991) to describe a public sector modernization wave. The NPM as a model for public sector reforms has spread rapidly to many countries. However, the effects of NPM are often promised or expected, but seldom much documented (Pollitt and Bouckaert, 2000).

The main hypothesis in the NPM reforms is that more market, more management and greater autonomy will produce more efficiency, without having negative side effects on other public sector values. However, tensions arise from a hybrid aspect of NPM. The tensions result from the contradiction between the *centralizing tendencies inherent in contractualism* (from economic organization theory) and the *devolutionary tendencies of managerialism* (from management theory). The paradigm in economic organization theory is that the power of political leaders must be reinforced against bureaucracy. This implies centralization, concentration of political power, co-ordination and control via contractual arrangements. The paradigm in management theory is that the primacy of managerial principles in bureaucracy must be re-established. However, enhancing the capacity of managers to take actions requires attention to decentralization, delegation and devolution, which must come into conflict with the political control and centralization prescribed by economic organization theory (Christensen and Lægreid, 2004: 13).

From the above presentation of NPM, we know the hybrid character of public sector reform. This hybrid character creates a tension between *contractualism* and *managerialism*, with the result that public sector organizations become more closed to their context, and more instrumental in their behaviour. However, in most countries, the NPM reforms have synthesized and adopted a blend of the two models. The countries have tried to give managers and their subordinates more autonomy and to strengthen political control through contracts, monitoring and incentive systems at the same time (Christensen and Lægreid, 2003). Reduced political control is the most significant consequence of NPM reform (Christensen and Lægreid, 2004; Pollitt and Bouckaert, 2000). There seems to be an anti-political trend that potentially can undermine political control, because devolution has increased the distance between the political leadership and the subordinate units and lower levels of management. There is a tendency to define political involvement in public enterprises as 'inappropriate' interference in business matters (Christensen and Lægreid, 2002).

An important consequence of these conflicting processes involves increased vertical and horizontal specialization and fragmentation. Authority is transferred downwards in the hierarchy, either between existing organizations or to new governmental organizations, both inside and outside the governmental administrative organization. The idea is to separate politics from administrative and commercial functions, and to make the public sector more like the private sector. This vertical specialization has often gone hand in hand with the horizontal specialization. Here, functions that were traditionally organized together, such as policy advice, regulative tasks, ownership functions, control functions and purchaser/provider functions, have now been separated into distinct units. Through this vertical and horizontal specialization, the NPM-modernized state has become more fragmented than the traditional integrated state model (Christensen and Lægreid, 2004: 15; Olsen, 1988).

Governance identifies the blurring of boundaries and responsibilities for tackling social and economic issues

Western societies suffer under instrumental rationalities and the neglect of communicative rationalities and collective process, and NPM reforms in the public sector seem to have enforced this process. It can be said that the situation in general is a consequence of the modernization process in our societies. In this process, instrumental rationality and top-down policy seem to dominate over communicative rationality and bottom-up policy. When this modern logic becomes dominant, strong professions and their respective sector authorities, which base their existence mainly on instrumental rationality, can achieve a strong position in society (Giddens, 1997; Habermas, 1995).

The NPM reforms intended to empower customers through free choice of services, to free managers from detailed political instructions, and to strengthen political steering through defining the long-term goals for the public sector and asserting the outcome (Christensen and Lægreid, 2003). However, these three intentions are difficult to achieve simultaneously (Pollitt and Bouckaert, 2000), and the consequence is a 'fragmentation of the national states' and an increased 'sector thinking and acting' (Christensen and Lægreid, 2004).

The NPM reforms seem to have freed managers from detailed political instructions, but have not strengthened the political steering because of the lack of causality in the production of public sector services. In public sector production, defining long-term and broadly accepted goals is difficult, and to establish obvious, logical relations between input and outcome is challenging. In addition, the monitoring and evaluation systems are, so far, more developed to handle *output* than *outcome*, because the lack of knowledge about the causalities between public sector activities and the results for society is enormous. In addition, every activity or every effect that can be measured tends to get most focus. Then, the nearest solution could be more monitoring, more evaluation and more accountability, but these activities do not solve the fundamental problem with the lack of causality in the production of public sector services. When there is no obvious, logical relation between a public sector organization activity, or lack of activity, and the outcome to the society, we cannot hold the organizations and their leaders responsible for the outcome.

Thus, the NPM reforms have delegated power from elected politicians to administrative leaders, with the consequence that the politicians are not able to hold the public sector managers responsible for the outcome of the policy implementation, only the output. We now tend to evaluate public and private sector leaders in much the same way, that is by their ability to lead their organizations to perform, measured by output indicators. This lack of *outcome accountability* gives the public sector managers the possibility to act in an egoistic way, and makes it extremely difficult to obtain outcome, such as sustainable public health, through the existing political and administrative sector structure. Therefore, there is a strong need for cross-sector networking, and public sector managers are expected to take part in partnerships and collaborative spatial planning and development at the same time as public sector organizations have become more instrumental and output-oriented. These network organizations are based on interdependency, trust and a mutual interest in achieving outcomes they cannot create alone. However, when silo thinking is dominant, the potential outcome from the partnership will always be compared with the transaction cost of staying in contact with the partners. The basic question for the participants seems to be '*what is in it for me?*' as a partner. As a consequence, NPM reform and the fragmentation of the political power structure actually have reduced the public sector's ability and willingness to participate in these network organizations, because the leaders have become more focused on internal issues and their production of output. Then, the nearest solution should be more accountability for public sector managers' production of outcome, but this is not a sufficient solution when the causality between long-term goals, input, output and outcome is vague. Today, the politicians get blamed when people do not like the outcome of public sector production, but the politicians are not able to hold the public sector managers responsible for the outcome of the policy implementation, only the output.

To empower customers through free choice of services is one of many forms of participation in policy-making and implementation, and can be a strong form of participation, if customers have alternatives to choose between. Citizen control over decisions is generally regarded as the most transformative and empowering form of participation. Arnstein (1969) defined a *ladder of citizen participation* stretching from citizen control as the strongest form, via delegated power, partnership, placation, consultation, to informing as the weakest form, and with therapy and manipulation as non-participation and the lowest rungs on the ladder. Many planners and researchers have experienced that even strong forms of participation do not necessarily challenge the established political power, as long as those in power can choose to take into account all the views expressed. This is particularly true for partnerships where the partners are not legally obligated to implement what they have agreed upon in the partnership. Many planners have also experienced that consultation is widely used in planning and development processes, both in organizations and communities, to legitimize decisions that have already been made.

Partnership and participation in planning emerged in the 1960s and have now become a part of the *communicative and collaborative turn* in planning (Healey, 1993). Broad participation in planning and development processes is now regarded as a necessity in order to achieve empowerment in communities. However, there is research that shows that participation in regional and local governance partnerships tends to become a professional, elite activity, involving employees from the public and private sectors rather than citizens and stakeholders (Swyngedouw, 2005).

Governance identifies the power dependence involved in the relationship between institutions involved in collective action

The bringing together of health with social and economic development has been a recent phenomenon. Barton and Tsourou (2000: 158) conclude, in their discussion on healthy urban planning (in a holistic sense), that, in European cities, planning is still largely conceptual, and many cities are working very traditionally, with disjointed sector activities, marginal projects and a short-term view of effects, especially in relation to economic benefits. However, an increasing number of cities are recognizing the link between health and urban planning, and they mention the WHO 'Healthy Cities' as evidence of an increasing level of collaboration between health and urban planning departments, not only for isolated projects, but in a strategic way.

Mobilizing for action through planning and partnership, which are the most recent tools in public health practice, is built upon a long history of planning by local public health agencies. Although the situation differs from country to country, most of the Western world is highly influenced by the planning approaches in the US. Here, public health planning has evolved over half a century from the earliest problem/programme-focused planning, through more comprehensive approaches, such as the Planned Approach to Community Health (PATCH) and the Assessment Protocol for Excellence in Public Health (APEXPH), to the strategic planning of today. Mobilizing for Action through Planning and Partnership (MAPP) introduces strategic thinking and system orientation into public health planning and builds upon this legacy (Lenihan, 2005). MAPP can be regarded as a concept that (Corso *et al.*, 2005: 388):

- supplements the APEXPH organizational capacity assessment indicators;
- expands the concept of community capacity to address the public health system, so as to recognize the contributions of all organizations in improving the community's health;
- adopts principles of strategic planning as the mechanism for focusing the resources and actions of the public health system; and
- creates a learning environment to generate an information flow among the work group, stakeholders, experts and others in recognition that success of a new practice tool would depend on it being firmly grounded in application experience.

Through MAPP, public health planning has evolved from the more traditional needs assessment and programme planning approaches, typically addressing single issues, to a model that is grounded in strategic planning concepts that try to put the most important issues on the agenda and to include new and diverse partners in the process. Closely related to this is dynamic systemic thinking, including feedback processes and the learning environment.

In the MAPP approach to planning, strategic planning evolves from a process that usually occurs within a single organization to one that occurs within an entire community. This reflects contemporary public health theory and practice. The effective response to public health outcomes needed in communities today requires collective action, and collective action requires both meaningful public health partnerships and an understanding of the resources in the community (Salem, 2005: 379). However, this new strategic approach to planning, which comes from the private sector, is not easily applied to the public sector (Bryson and Roering, 1987).

To illustrate this effort to apply private sector strategic planning approaches to the public sector, we will use regional planning in Norway as an example. Here, we find an important and interesting difference between sectoral and territorial policies, and this difference is most clearly expressed in the two forms of regional planning (R. Amdam, 2002).

1   *Planning in regional organizations (sectoral regional planning)*
    The first form is sectoral regional planning, which, in the main, is
    planning and development work that is restricted to the public service
    production areas that are the responsibility of agencies, municipalities and
    counties. In effect, this is the planning and implementation of welfare
    state service productions in regionalized organizations. This is a form of
    activity planning that has many common features with private and
    voluntary sector planning. To the extent that these organizations refer
    to this form of planning as regional planning, we would characterize it
    as a sector-dominated and fragmented, top-down policy-implementing
    form of regional planning.

2   *Planning in the regional society (territorial regional planning)*
    The second form is the territorial regional planning that is carried out,
    to a large extent, across municipalities and counties and is concerned
    with spatial development and themes such as industrial development,
    transport, communications, land-use planning and co-operation in the
    production of services. It is typical of this planning that, in addition to
    including municipalities and counties, it also attempts to involve other
    public authorities, as well as the private and voluntary sectors, in forms
    of partnership in planning and implementation. The actual regional
    planning would thus appear to take place, to a great extent, in formal
    network organizations between delegates/representatives from the
    public, private and voluntary sectors and from the various levels of
    government. This is a cross-sector and territorial, bottom-up policy-
    making form of regional planning.

The first form of planning is mainly a part of a top-down regime
dominated by central planning and control of welfare state production. The
second is mainly a part of a territorial, bottom-up regime of mobilization,
innovation and competition between regions. Until recently, these regimes
were integrated in the municipalities and counties, but, today, municipalities
and counties engage in the new regional governance structures and processes
because of the rigidity of the top-down government structures and the
flexibility of the governance structures. They set up partnerships between
the public, private and voluntary sectors in order to influence policy outside
the direct control of the local government structure.

The sectoral planning in municipalities and counties has the main focus
on their part of the welfare state production, and the territorial planning
in inter-municipality and inter-county institutions has a focus on society as
a whole. As a consequence, the two planning systems seem to get more and
more separated, and this process is 'learning-by-doing' driven. These are
processes that are known from other countries (see, for example, Zoete,
2000). The two-parallel system of regional planning seems to become both
logical and desirable. It becomes logical that territorial regional planning,
which, in general, emphasizes spatial development and innovation, in the

main is carried out in informal network organizations based on the public, private and voluntary sectors; and, moreover, that sector-based regional planning, which, in general, is planning of sector activities, is carried out within the domains of the formal government organizations, but that this planning both receives and delivers premises for territorial planning. Or, to put it another way, the challenge of territorial regional planning is to get organizations in the public, private and voluntary sectors to participate in the one or more network organizations or partnerships that the territorial regional planning manages to establish.

Thus, territorial regional planning needs to become an institutional capacity-building process (Healey, 1997; 1999). The local and regional planning and development organizations must be regarded as legitimate and have to be accepted by the public, private and voluntary sectors, and by local, regional and national levels of government. In contrast to the sector organizations, these territorial partnership organizations cannot (will not) be given legitimacy from a superior institution in the political power structure, because none seems to have the full and necessary cross-sector legitimacy in relation to regional planning and development work. Local and regional political agencies have to create their legitimacy through their work, that is, in a political will-formation process (Habermas, 1995).

Governance is about autonomous, self-governing networks of actors

It seems to be commonly recognized that public health work is about multi-actor and multilevel empowerment approaches, including governmental policies and actions in the legal, economic and political arenas. It is about coalitions and inter-sectoral partnership between academic institutions, government agencies, NGOs and communities. Thus, building and sustaining formal and informal networks become necessary for maintaining relationship and communication channels. If public health leaders do not view net-working as an ongoing and essential activity in the agency's operation, they may find that once-useful communication channels no longer exist when they are needed. The key to successful networks is identifying and assessing the network structure that is in place and understanding the effect of the structure on available resources in public health (Nicola and Hatcher, 2000: 6).

Policy rhetoric promoting a broad partnership is now a cornerstone in public health work; however, it can be argued that a good partnership depends on limiting the number of parties in the collaborative process. The number of members cannot be so great that the process of partnership becomes unmanageable. The process of partnership must be inclusive as well as exclusive. In addition, a great number of parties being involved in the partnerships makes the complexity of accountability higher. In different partnership working, considerable thought has been given to ensuring an open and transparent process, but still, ensuring accountability across organizational boundaries remains a sensitive area (Asthana *et al.*, 2002).

Government and governance can both be characterized by their ability to make decisions and their capacity to enforce them. The main difference between them is that organizations within government rest on resources under the authority and sanction of the government. Governance is the creation of a structure that cannot be externally imposed but is the outcome of the interaction of influencing actors in a multi-actor system. For governance, the ultimate partnership activity is to form a self-governing network (Stoker, 1998: 23). The emerging governance forms are highly context-dependent and located in specific institutional dynamics. However, the NPM reform is a worldwide process that makes public and voluntary organizations become more like private sector organizations, with a dominance of instrumental rationality and internal focus. In addition, the lack of outcome accountability gives public sector organizations the possibility to act in an egoistic way and makes it extremely difficult to realize local and regional territorial planning and development through governance and network organizations that require altruistic actions. This situation can actually reduce the existing and potential power of governance and partnership activity, because the creation of these is very dependent on trust between the participants and willingness to support the production of common good. If we regard governance as a government response to the fragmentation of the state, and if the government institutions have become more egoistic, Jessop (1997) may be correct when he writes that governance still seems to exist in the shadow of government.

The term *network organizations* can be used as a collective term for partnership and governance in regional planning and development, which covers multilevel and multi-sector co-operation, such as governing bodies that are comprised of actors from the vertical and the horizontal power structures. The term network organization covers a collaboration of organizations of various types (Strand, 2001: 267). Common to all of them is the fact that the collaborating organizations can have a large degree of independence, and that they, to a great extent, can disappear from the network, either of their own free will, or because the partners choose to exclude them.

Actors in network organizations gain capacity to act by blending their resources, skills and purpose into a long-term coalition. Network organizations are therefore complex and dissolvable. They are *complex* because they are made up of organizations that are quite different, but that contribute to the network with their own speciality. They are *dissolvable* in the sense that participating organizations can be replaced, and the network itself can have its strength completely disbanded.

Network organizations are often regarded as more innovative and able to handle uncertainty than bureaucratic organizations, but this ought to be handled more as a hypothesis than axiomatic fact (Olsen, 2004). However, network organizations are normally loosely coupled organizations, and therefore obtain the power and legitimacy the different collaborating organizations want to give them, and the power the context can accept (Strand, 2001).

Participation in network organizations may be motivated by self-interest or on the basis of mutual usefulness and common values, and the collaboration is normally formalized through agreements and transaction control mechanisms between the participants. In theory, the control mechanism in network organizations can be based on market, bureaucracy or trust (Langfield-Smith and Smith, 2003: 286). However, accountability deficits do often become a problem, because network organizations have a significant degree of autonomy and are driven by the self-interest of their members, rather than a wider concern with the public interest or, particularly, those excluded from the network (Stoker, 1998: 24).

Network organizations in regional planning and development can be understood as *interactive governance* based on partnership between actors across government levels and government sectors (Veggeland, 2000). This means that the partnerships become a political arena in the intersection between vertical and horizontal power, and between functional and territorial logic, but not in such a way that one dominates the other. If the power imbalance becomes a pattern, the losing actors in the network organizations will respond by withdrawing, and the multidimensional policy will fall apart. Here, we find one of the greatest challenges facing governance-based regional planning. This challenge is at the very core of the modernization of society and is associated with the comprehensive and serious criticism that, in modern society, vertical and instrumental logic dominates horizontal and communicative logic.

Local and regional development agencies as network organizations operate initially in environments that are typical for trust-based transactions, that is, the control mechanism is characterized by low levels of task programmability and low levels of output measurability. The initial selection of partners is based on perceptions of trust that arise through friendship, former contractual relationships and reputation. The contracts are broad frameworks that tend to become more detailed over time. The context is complex and changing, and the performance has low repetitiveness. Contracts tend to grow out of the need for formalization of co-operation. However, problems can arise when the participating organizations, which are most familiar with market-based (private sector) and bureaucracy-based (public sector) transaction control mechanisms, form powerful network organizations based on trust. These problems have potentially arisen with the NPM reforms, because the reforms seem to have transformed public sector organizations away from trust-based relationships to more *mistrust-based* transactions.

The *legitimacy* of network organizations is, to all intents and purposes, dependent on the *productivity* and *efficiency* they can demonstrate, and to what degree the actual process justifies their existence. Hence, the legitimacy of such an organization will come both from inside and outside. The legitimacy from within will depend on how much power the participating organizations are willing to transfer to the network, and this transfer is normally limited by what is in the interests of the participant at any time. In understanding the acceptance and legitimacy from outside, it is important to stress the fact that network organizations will be involved in a continual competition with other organizations, and that they will challenge the power in the vertical and horizontal power structures in the society. It is therefore vital for the legitimacy of network organizations that the participating organizations act in the networks with powers of attorney that are well supported in their organizations.

Stoker (2004: 27) talks about *'network community governance'* as an emerging new form of management. He concludes, in his discussion, that network community governance marks a break from traditional public administration and NPM in its vision of the role of local government and its understanding of the context for governing and the core process of governance. In network community governance, the overarching goal is greater effectiveness in tackling the problems that the public sector most cares about; no one sector has the monopoly on the public sector ethos, and relationships are maintained through shared values. This new network governance is seemingly a return to a more value-based governance and a restoration of core public sector values, such as separated powers, democracy, transparency, accountability, equity and effectiveness.

Governance recognizes the capacity to get things done that does not rest on the power of government to command and use its authority

Friedmann (1992) claims that the modernization has led to an increased emphasis on instrumental rationality and the promoting of self-interest, and that the process has a negative effect on communicative common sense, which, in the main, is kept alive in the democratic governing bodies and in civil society. He maintains that politics should lead to the formation of a moral fellowship, and that political activity cannot therefore be reduced to the economic calculation of utilitarian values and sociological determinism. However, Friedmann himself is aware that the strengthening of relations between civil society and the people's democratically elected representatives often meets strong opposition from the established government structure. Seen in relation to local and regional planning and public health work, this will involve strengthening planning's territorial dimension at the expense of the sector dimension. To put it another way, cross-sector co-ordination can only be achieved by creating a collective territorial counterbalance to the vertical and sector-based governance structure.

This territorial collective counterforce can be regarded as a *community capacity-building process*, a process based on the principle of empowerment. According to the World Bank, two attributes of empowerment are articulated in this process:

1   the role of agencies of marginal communities to exercise choice and transform their lives; and
2   the role of opportunity structure, the institutional, political, economic and governmental context that either allows actors to create effective actions or inhibits them.

Empowerment cannot be given to people or done to people, but comes from processes where people empower themselves. External change agents may catalyse actions or help create arenas for people to learn, but empowerment occurs only if people create their own momentum, gain their own skills and advocate their own changes. Collective action is regarded as being dependent on three stages:

1   the political, economic, social, informational and moral bases from which people start;
2   the communities' individual skills and collective action capacity; and
3   the results people are able to obtain.

In addition, empowerment processes may lead to challenges of powerful forces, including governmental institutions. Local, state and national government, as major players in the opportunity structure, must have a focus on empowerment strategies that force improved responsiveness to constituents and enhance transparency, uncorrupted government, greater efficiency and more equitable distribution of resources and services to communities (HEN, 2006: 19).

Nicola and Hatcher (2000) discuss a framework and guidance on building effective public health constituencies to achieve community health improvement, and compare different planning approaches from a leadership perspective. They write that knowing the community is essential, because social programmes tend to fail owing to a lack of appropriate management and an oversimplified view of constituent motivation. They argue that knowing the community and its constituents is more than epidemiological assessment, and, if public health leaders view networking as an ongoing and essential activity in the agency's operations, constituency mobilization can be productive and require minimal efforts. Wilson (2004: 409) argues that national health programmes need to be structured in a way that balances the advantages of regional approaches to public health challenges with the benefits of a co-ordinated central response, and the policy-makers need to address the unique challenges of public health governance.

Politically strong and economically dynamic local and regional communities are often characterized by people participating in both professional and local networks, and by the integration of local horizontal and global vertical relationships. Many researchers see the community with a strong civil society and a strong democratic process as the main key to dynamic regional development (see, among others, Bennett and McCoshan, 1993; Dryzek, 1990; Forester, 1993; Friedmann, 1992; Putnam, 1993; Stöhr, 1990; and Storper, 1997). However, development work based on instrumental rationality is concentrated on strengthening the vertical power structure through seeking for cost-effective organization and maximized utilization of resources. This kind of development process can lead to bigger regional dependency on national-level institutions and large companies. It can also weaken the local communities' capability to learn and to handle challenges (Giddens, 1997; Habermas, 1984; 1987; 1995; Stöhr, 1990).

From this perspective, it becomes logical to empower regional and local communities to oppose the dominant vertical and instrumental power structure (Friedmann and Weaver, 1979). This involves a strengthening of the horizontal power structure through activating civil society, the elected representatives, and through local embedding of private businesses. In this way, horizontal political power can be organized to supplement and oppose the sector-dominated and vertical power structure. However, dynamic local and regional communities cannot be seen as units that are more or less independent of central government and external companies. Nor are regions and communities that lag behind necessarily units that are strongly dependent on superior governing institutions and external enterprises. The promotion of a regional development requires that the region itself take more responsibility for its development as a political actor (Keating, 1996). This regional drive to create *competitive advantages* from place to place has the inevitable logic that there will be winners and losers (Dunford, 1994). Thus, the regions have a strong need for *regional political institutions* that can work on a collective level to promote the region's needs, interests and values in the mainly political power structure where the different sectors' knowledge and actions dominate.

In this perspective, *regions* are not a fixed structure, and regional *institutional capacity building* is a process (Healey, 1999; 2001; Paasi, 1986). Regimes, partnerships, networks and coalitions have to be constructed and managed (Amin and Thrift, 1995). Regions need a well-developed 'institutional thickness', understood as the totality of social, cultural and institutional forms and supports available to entrepreneurs and organizations. This includes trade associations, voluntary agencies, sectoral coalitions and local elites, their common agreements, shared views and interpretations, and their effects on local policy. Thus, the new regional political institutions need a political process to make them legitimate political actors. Historically, the term *region as a political actor* has been used in two connections (Baldersheim, 2000; Keating, 1996):

1   In a top-down tradition, regions are a part of the nation-building process and a means to decentralize power and responsibility to territories within the nation. Rokkan and Urwin (1983) talk about four phases in this process: territorial consolidation, cultural standardizing, democratization and creation of a welfare state.

2   In a bottom-up tradition, the regions are arenas for social mobilization. According to Paasi (1986: 121), this is an institution-building process. Elements or phases in this process are: localization of organized social practices; formation of identity; emergence of institutions; and the achievement of administrative status as an established spatial structure.

According to Paasi *et al.* (1994), a region represents the condensation of a complex history of economic, political and social processes into a specific cultural image. Central to Paasi's analysis is the institutionalization of the region, defined as the socio-spatial process during which some territorial units emerge as part of the spatial structure of a society and become established and clearly identified in the distinct spheres of social action and social consciousness (Paasi, 1986: 121). As a consequence, a legitimate regional political institution in the new regional policy must be a fruitful combination of nation building and local mobilization, of top-down and bottom-up politics, of government and governance, and of instrumental and communicative rationality.

Conclusions

In a regional policy context, this means that the bottom-up, mainly communicative power is used to equalize the top-down, mainly instrumental power and to build adequate local and regional development institutions. This can be called the governance turn in regional planning, but, in practice, the new governance structure seems to exist in the shadow of the old governance structure. In fact, local and regional planning and development more and more seem to take the form of a two-parallel system: (1) government-dominated, highly sectorized and single-organization planning and (2) governance-based spatial planning that tries to foster collaboration and partnership. Regional development agencies are the key actors in spatial planning, but they are often rather weak constructions that depend greatly on the trust between the participants in the agencies, their willingness to collaborate and their commitment to local and regional development.

As far as we can draw conclusions from our discussion, there seems to be a similar governance turn in public health work, and the experiences from this turn seem to be similar to the experiences from regional policy. A common and overall experience is that governance is a complicated process. In order to make a territorial counterforce to the sectorized power that dominates modern societies, partnerships in public health, as well as local and regional development, need to create legitimacy from inside the community and achieve acceptance and legitimacy from outside. Then, our conclusion becomes a kind of dilemma. Partnerships within the governance structure need to be strong enough to influence their partners from the government structure, but is that possible in governance-based partnerships, where the participants from the government structure are free to leave? Handling this dilemma is at the core of what policy-making is about.

Habermas's (1995) contribution to this discussion is the concept of *political will-formation processes*, based on dialogues between participants in the public sphere where there is a balance of power and where the pressure to state one's reasons is present. Inspired by Habermas's political will-formation process and our own research in the field of regional planning and development, we have constructed a political legitimating planning process called empowerment planning (R. Amdam, 1997c; 2001; 2004). We will present this model in the next chapter.

3 Planning in regional development and public health work

An empowerment model

In this chapter, we present the empowerment-planning model that was introduced for the HEPRO partners on several occasions, and that was an important part of the training programme for the partners. The model has been developed over a long period and is based on our action research in neighbourhoods, municipalities, and local and regional communities. The action research process has had the same characteristics as what we, in Chapter 1, called the epistemology of social practice. The model took form in a combination of radical practice and critical reflections and is well documented in my doctoral thesis (R. Amdam, 1997a; 1997b). In this chapter, we will introduce some of the theoretical foundations of the model and we will outline the model as it was presented for the HEPRO project.

Introduction

With the turn from government to governance comes the need for a different form of planning. When the state has a strong role as a major developer of society and communities, the government institutions have the legitimacy to conduct instrumental and mainly top-down master planning. This form of planning is fitted to solve many of the problems the planning faces, as far as we are talking about the formation of governmental, top-down and sectorized public services provision. However, planning is not just about forming policies and programmes, but also about implementing these through collective actions. A common critique of instrumental, top-down planning is that neither the plan nor the implementation is embedded in local and regional institutions. These plans are usually drawn up by experts, without broad participation. As we have argued in Chapters 1 and 2, in the governance structure, communicative planning is a prerequisite for building partnerships between the private, public and voluntary sectors, and between local, regional, national and international levels. In the planning literature, there is a growing understanding that the main challenge is not to choose between instrumental and communicative planning and between top-down and bottom-up approaches, but how to integrate them in the practice of empowerment. From our point of view, the policy will-forming process or communicative action theory represents one very promising way of integrating them (see Chapter 1).

Empowerment planning

The term 'empowerment' is a complicated idea. Empowerment implies a gathering of power, in a dynamic way, over a period of time. One way of becoming empowered is the transfer of power from the top down, involving an empowerer and those empowered. Another way is where power is created from the bottom up, by somebody who previously perceived him- or herself to be powerless. This distinction is parallel to *top-down and bottom-up policy*, *exogenous and indigenous development*, and *instrumental and communicative rationality*. From the discussion in Chapters 1 and 2, we now know that, in empowerment practice, there is a strong need to combine the top-down and bottom-up approaches, and we seem to need practical and tested planning models that show us that the combination of top down and bottom up is possible in practice.

Bottom-up planning, as an alternative approach to traditional, top-down planning, places the emphasis on direct democracy, autonomy in the decision-making of territorially organized communities, local self-reliance and experiential social learning. Its starting point is the locality, because *civil society* is most readily mobilized around local issues. Civil society is the many-standard order that arises from those values and interests that are shared by most of the people in particular communities. The aim is to mobilize civil society and transfer the social power to political power. In this way, local and regional planning becomes a process of institutional capacity building (Healey, 1999).

In our analyses of the institutionalization of regions in the Norwegian context, we have found it fruitful to separate sectoral planning from territorial planning. The first is mainly a part of a top-down regime dominated by central planning and control of the welfare state production. The second is mainly a part of a territorial, bottom-up regime of mobilization, innovation and competition between regions. *Sectoral regional planning* is an integrated part of the top-down, nation-building process and the government structure, and is regarded as legitimate when it provides technical and economic efficiency seen from the different sectors. For *territorial regional planning*, the situation is different. This is mainly a bottom-up, institution-building process based on social mobilization and governance (R. Amdam, 2002). In many ways, territorial planning will come to oppose and challenge sectoral planning and power, but territorial planning will not generate more legitimacy than the process itself can create and the sectorized national authorities want to give planning. As a consequence, territorial regional planning becomes very dependent on acceptance from the national state authorities. As far as we know, this two-parallel planning system is not a particular issue for Norway. With reference to the Netherlands, Hajer and

Zonneveld (2000) argue in favour of a 'societal turn' in planning in order to handle the network society. Their alternative is to allow regions greater autonomy in a system of spatial development planning, and make the national government more selective in its involvement.

Consequently, it is important that the planner not only has knowledge of planning as a tool, but also knows the political reality in which the tool is to be used. Planners who lack the necessary insight into the political structure, culture and processes can make mistakes that lead both the planner and the planning into a state of discredit. This statement seems to count also for public health promoters. Laverack and Labonte (2000: 255) discuss their role in empowerment work and they conclude that there has been little clarification of how to make the concept of empowerment operational in public health work. Let us, therefore, look a bit closer at the signs of political processes, before we go further into the design of the empowerment-planning model.

Jacobsen (1964) has given a *definition of politics* that has been much used, which is in line with Pollitt and Bouckaert (2000) and Lukes (1974), and which we presented in Chapter 1. Jacobsen writes that politics can be seen as an activity that evolves around finding ways of formulating problems, trying to get these formulations accepted as binding and eventually organizing continuous problem-solving activities around these problems (see Figure 3.1). In comparison with this, Lundquist (1976) has defined *planning* as a futuristic process where the actors seek to achieve control over their surroundings so that, through this, they can achieve their intentions.

If we see planning as a tool in the political process, which Jacobsen defines, the challenge will be to get the problems accepted and then organize actions so that the problems can be solved in a futuristic and intended way. Thus, both politics and planning evolve around having the power to promote wishes, interests and values. However, great uncertainty about the future, due to the complexity and the pace of change in modern society, has led to

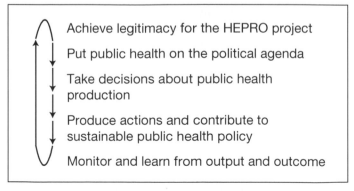

Figure 3.1 Public health planning is a policy process

a lack of trust in rational calculations as a model for decisions, and has moved the attention over to models that are based on communication and learning (Sager, 1990). This change also affects the view of planning and leads to essential changes in the relationship between planning and politics. In instrumental planning models based on rational calculations, it is, in theory, possible to separate politics and planning. Thus, planning can be separated into a subject-independent activity based on preparing political decisions. However, communicative planning is based on the presumption that the present and the future are being formed in inter-subjective learning processes between actors, and the planner becomes one of many actors contributing to the process. Thus, most people will see the planner and the other participants in the planning process as political actors, with their own values, needs and interests (Flyvbjerg, 1993; 1996).

When we say that planning and politics can be divided, we can easily fall into the trap of seeing planning as something positive, because we believe that it is logical and functional. In addition, we can see the forming of politics as something negative, because we see it as illogical and dysfunctional (Minogue, 1993: 20). Offerdal (1992) wrote that, in order to maintain a positive presumption of the structuring of politics and the *politicians*, the process of politics must be underlined. By this, he means that there are political ways of solving a problem that are necessary for us to be able to maintain a society and a type of government that provide each individual with an opportunity to take part in the governing and, at the same time, be able to act as an independent individual. Politics is using common principles in concrete situations, which gives the politicians both freedom and responsibility and, consequently, the opportunity to learn on different levels. Thus, Offerdal maintains that politicians have a certain expertise that is often necessary in all stages of the controlling process within a political governing system, and that is not only occupied with establishing objectives. Offerdal (1992) writes further that politics is not the fixed, calculating approach that is being demanded by instrumental rationality. However, it seems as though politics, in many ways, is being coloured by this way of thinking and acting, and this makes politics apolitical or unpolitical. With this label, he means politics where the actions that are initiated on behalf of society are argued for with focus on what is necessary (faith, facts, expertise or other types of 'tyrant'). Consequently, he claims that proper political processes and institutions need democratically elected people who, through dialogue and negotiation, can try to unite differing values, interests and needs.

Political institutions and institution building

According to Olsen (1988), a *political institution* in government or governance is a structure between the individual and society. The structure is not a neutral mirror of micro-motives or macro-forces, but modifies and is modified by both forces. The structure manages authority and power, but also collective wisdom, ethics and norms, and shows the signs of a certain political order (March and Olsen, 1976). Institutions create order in behaviour and ways of thinking, but they are still temporary and limited forms of order. Political institutions are part of the political process, and, over time, the institution itself will exercise a conservative power by defining which actors, problems, solutions and deciding factors are to be recognized as legitimate. The political institutions can be separated from community and society and become a sort of filter between the organization and its context. It is, therefore, important that political institutions are subject to a completely open public scrutiny, so that citizens can monitor what the institutions are doing. The separation of political institutions from community and society can only be counteracted by a strengthening of democracy and transparency, through media coverage, open hearings, public meetings, and so on. Here, we see the importance of what Habermas describes as the *public sphere* (Habermas, 1984; 1987). When citizens meet to discuss collectively relevant questions or to act together, they develop a communicative power that can, and should, exert influence on the political system.

As we have written above, we consider Habermas's work on discursive will formation a flexible and promising guide to future institutional reforms (Habermas, 1995). In this work, he argues in favour of combining instrumental and communicative rationality in an open, policy-legitimizing process (see Chapter 1). In this will-forming process, Habermas presents different discourses with their respective rationalities; together, these form a political legitimizing process. Habermas understands the political process as a will-formation process starting with pragmatic discourses, which further lead to ethical and moral discourses, depending on the kinds of conflict present. These discourses can lead to juridical discourses, which are concerned with the degree of consistency in laws and regulations. Procedure-regulated negotiation can be an alternative to discourses, if the latter do not produce sufficient consensus.

The discursive process is conducted by means of public argumentation. It is through public debate among free citizens that proposals can be justified or legitimated. Communicative rationality can contribute to building morality-forming communities and to integrating individual and collective values, interests and needs. In the political will-formation process, instrumental rationality, with its focus on facts and truth, meets with communicative rationality, with its focus on sincerity and comprehensibility. Facts and truth usually depend on paradigmatic values, morality and views. Therefore, communicative rationality has to be made superior to instrumental rationality (Dryzek, 1990; Friedmann, 1992; Habermas, 1995).

Habermas (1995) claims that, in undistorted discourses, *equal power* and the *duty to argue* for whatever claims you make are prerequisites. For undistorted discourses, *validity claims* have been made that imply that the speech acts are to be tested for their *truthfulness, sincerity, rightness* and *comprehensibility*. The duty to argue, together with the demand for public transparency, forces the participants to provide their statements with a defence, even towards citizens who are not presently part of the discourse. The weightiest argument will, ideally, be given the most weight in the process of creating consensus. However, the outcome may well be, and often is, a compromise or a major decision. A legitimate decision does not represent the will of all, but is one that results from the deliberation of all (Manin, 1987: 352).

In our understanding of Habermas's political will-forming or legitimating process, *juridical discourse* concerns the rules of juridical consistency. This is planning as a systematic process of developing a frame of reference for future decisions and actions by a relevant community. These issues concern the relationship between the context and the planning institution, and the normative influence of the formally decided planning documents and other juridical norms. This discourse is about the mission, acceptance and legitimacy, and is the topic of what we call *institutional planning*.

Moral discourse concerns the conflicts of norms and values, and is a topic for mainly communicative planning, that is, planning as a social, interactive process between actors who are seeking consensus and mutual understanding. These are questions that are the issues for mobilizing and for *strategic planning*.

Ethical–political discourse involves a discussion of whose needs, interests and values are to be favoured. Conflicts of interests are often connected with the utilization of resources in co-ordinative planning, that is, planning with the focus on how to deploy organizations to undertake the necessary actions at the appropriate time to accomplish mutually agreed-upon outcomes. This discourse refers to the questions of organization, co-ordination and *tactical planning*.

Pragmatic discourse concerns the discussion of facts and data and is a discourse tied mainly to instrumental rationality, that is, planning as a deliberative activity of problem-solving, involving rational choices by self-interested individuals or homogenous social units. The objective of rational planning is for the actors to decide to what ends future actions should be undertaken, and what course of action would be most effective. These elements are at the core of implementation and *operative planning*.

Adapting the legitimating model to planning

In several of our works, we have adapted Habermas's model of political will formation to a model for regional and local planning and development by establishing links between the development variables in regional development processes and the planning tools that are relevant in regional planning (see J. Amdam and R. Amdam, 2000; R. Amdam, 1997a; 1997b; 1997c; 2001; 2002; 2005).

We sum up the existing research by claiming that regional and local planning and development processes depend upon the existence of an appropriate balance between five variables: context, mobilization, organization, implementation and learning (see Figure 3.2). In the model, the five variables are linked together in an institution-building process that is dependent on all the elements. The model tells us which variables we should try to stimulate if we wish to promote empowerment. This message seems to have a generally strong statement, making it count for regions and communities that already have strong institutional capacity and dynamic processes, as well as for those that have potential capacity and dynamic processes. This implies that we can use the model in both explanatory and normative models.

In addition, we have experienced that a strategic planning approach, with institutional, strategic, tactical and operative levels, combined with a monitoring and evaluation process, seems to be a good concept for stimulating the five variables in development work at local, municipal and regional level (see Figure 3.3).

However, in accordance with the theory presented here, our research shows that, when this planning system is used, communicative rationality must be dominant compared with instrumental rationality. Instrumental rationality can be used in situations where the problem is technical, the climate is consensus, and the process is controlled (Gunsteren, 1976). This implies that instrumental rationality can be used at the operative level, but only if the institutional, strategic and tactical planning based on communicative rationality has succeeded in reducing the uncertainty of the situation down to the level needed for instrumental rationality (R. Amdam, 1997a; 1997b).

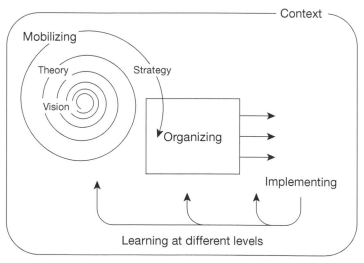

Figure 3.2 Development variables

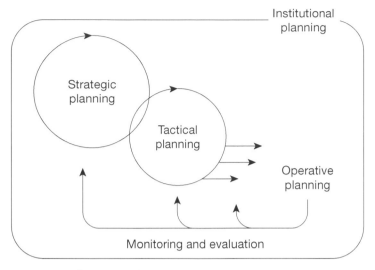

Figure 3.3 Planning tools

Our model can be summarized in three statements:

- *Statement 1*: Planning is about political power and policy-making (see Figure 3.1).
- *Statement 2*: Development processes have five variables (see Figure 3.2).
- *Statement 3*: Planning is the tool to stimulate the variables (see Figure 3.3).

Juridical discourse, institutional planning and context

Juridical discourse concerns the actual legitimacy and consistency of the rules of law. It also includes the planning documents' normative effect in relation to other plans and to rules of law, norms, regulations and guidelines for governing society. For all political institutions, this is one of the fundamental dimensions, because it really concerns the reason for their existence. For established institutions, this involves resisting the pressure from their surroundings for change in well-established structures, processes and cultures (Olsen, 1988).

In regional policy and theory, there is a growing awareness of the need for regional empowerment between the forces of globalization and internationalization at the supranational level, and the forces of mobilization and innovation at the regional and local levels. One characteristic of empowered regions and communities is that extensive communicative and collaborative partnerships between the public, private and voluntary sectors exist, both inside and outside the geographical territory. This does not mean that empowered regions and communities are units that are more or less independent of instrumental power from the superior government and external enterprises, and that lagging regions are units that are strongly dependent on support from the national government and external enterprises. In practice, all regions and communities are dependent on a widespread interaction with their surroundings, but the balance of power can easily become asymmetric. The achievement of an appropriate balance of power between the regions and communities and their surroundings is probably one of the most difficult tasks in local and regional development work. Both private enterprises and public governments can easily become too instrumental and top-down oriented and, thus, send the region into a *dependency relationship* (Friedmann, 1992; Friedmann and Weaver, 1979). This kind of dependency relationship can imply that actors outside the region take important decisions and actions regarding the region, and that people in the region are not actively involved in the social learning and mobilizing process. In this way, local and regional communities can enter a vicious circle that, over time, can weaken their own capability for facing new challenges, and they get what can be called *local community AIDS* (Stöhr, 1990: 2).

Empowered local and regional communities have, seemingly, an administrative limitation or a geographical limitation. However, such a view misses out the fact that these local and regional communities often are empowered and dynamic because they have both a territorial and a functional extent, combined with a strong identity. This implies that we need to take into account the character of communities, such as history and context, when we design regional planning and development interventions. Regional and local development is a slow, organic process. It takes root slowly and has to be carefully nurtured before it begins to yield results. Friedmann (1987) claims that local development cannot be organized and supported by authority bases in the society, but has to grow from within local communities. However, planners who come from the outside can, among other things, help to develop a new self-understanding and improve skills in self-help, direct action, negotiating and drawing up effective plans of action to achieve changes in policy processes and structures.

In regional and local planning and development work, the responsibility for actions is divided between many organizations and between government levels, and the work is often organized as programmes and projects similar to the HEPRO project. Therefore, there is a need for a partnership between the actors, but the establishment of these partnerships requires that the actors are able to commit themselves to co-operative networks or formal organizations. We will use *institutional partnerships* as a term for these partnerships, and by this we mean judicially binding agreements that regulate the responsibilities between the actors for implementing the programme or project. Institutional partnership is highly formalized, has an external given acceptance and legitimacy, and a limited number of members. The main purpose of these networks is frame setting for other partnerships, and, in practice, these partnerships are superior to other partnerships. In a project, the steering group will have the character of an institutional partnership.

The process of establishing these partnerships is a systematic process for developing a frame of reference for future decisions and actions. We call this process *institutional planning*, and, for partnerships, it involves obtaining power in practical politics and achieving an accepted and legitimate position in the system of governance.

Essentially, institutional planning concerns the relationships between the community and the structural powers in a context that creates both opportunities and obstacles for the local and regional communities as political actors. The degree of emphasis on actors and structures in empirical and theoretical research varies. In our works, we emphasize the mutual relationships between them, in line with Giddens (1984) and others. In concrete terms, this means that the building up of an institutional capacity in a region takes place in interaction with the region's surroundings. Therefore, planning must attempt to bring to light structural forces in the context and find out to what extent they represent opportunities or threats for the community. Furthermore, we must look at the power in the region's learning process, and to what extent this learning process transforms people's values, interests and actions. This means that actor–structure relationships also become important for the other discourses in Habermas's model of political will formation.

We usually organize the planning and development effort in regional and local communities as a project with a steering group as the co-ordinating body, and we often set up a team for teaching, supervision and evaluation. The main purpose of the project is to set up planning that stimulates mobilizing, organizing, implementing and learning processes in the community, and to produce plan documents with institutional, strategic, tactical, operative and evaluating content. However, the local process will usually not give the process and plan sufficient legitimacy. There will be a need for formal decisions in several institutions in the superior political power structure. Local and regional planning exists in the interface between actors from both the vertical and horizontal power structures; the different actors are in the special situation of needing approval and legitimacy from both structures. That is, from the governing levels: municipality, county and state; and from the governing systems: voluntary, private and public sectors, including democratically elected representatives. In practical planning, this implies that the planning process must incorporate actors from both the horizontal and vertical structures, and that the planning documents must be formally accepted in the appropriate organizations that belong to the two structures.

It is important to emphasize that regional and local planning and development work can be intensified by way of a project, but that it is nonetheless a continuous process. Organizing development work as a project can be a useful method of approach when an all-out effort is required, for a limited period, in a limited area. A well-established project presupposes that the members of the steering group have arrived at a reasonable degree of agreement about aims and means and, not least, about the limits of, and the mandate for, the project. Without the clarification of such questions, internal conflicts within the steering group can paralyse the whole project. It is also vital that the participants, as far as possible, enjoy equal rights when it comes to the terms of participation.

Moral discourses, strategic planning and mobilization

The moral discourse concerns norm conflicts and fundamental values and whose needs and values are to be favoured. This activity may also be referred to as a consensus-building activity (Healey, 1997; Innes *et al.*, 1994) and may involve developing a broad common understanding of development features and challenges and visions of what situation one desires and strategies for achieving this situation. In other words, agree on a political agenda (Lukes, 1974) and build up a collective capacity for action. This is at the core of mobilization and strategic planning.

If several people share the same values and act in a roughly similar fashion, this will form the foundation for a strong *identity* and a regional or local *culture*, in the form of a *moral collective* that defines its duties and rights. However, in order to achieve this culture, open democratic arenas are necessary where people can meet both for the exchange of views and for political action. In order to build such moral-forming collectives, it is important that the people participate as citizens who are concerned with the common good, and not as calculating experts in their field who are only intent on advancing their own interests. Therefore, strong and active civil societies and social networks are decisive arenas for building moral collectives (see, among others, Putnam, 1993). Moral collectives help to create the trust between people that is necessary to encourage them to make a stand for the collective, without fear of being exploited by persons who are simply out to promote their own interests, without considering the consequences for the collectives of which they are a part.

By mobilization, we mean strengthening the local and regional communities' activity to improve political capacity by stimulating the mutual understanding of their own situation and challenges, and of how the communities can work to achieve common goals. This involves focusing attention on structures and processes in the community, and on relationships between the local and regional community and society at large, and it means that the community must clarify how to work to influence these elements and relationships. For this reason, we stress the importance of strengthening the general understanding by establishing new arenas that allow the local inhabitants and other important actors to meet across the traditional boundaries of political administrative levels, administrative systems and political interests, regardless of personal characteristics such as age, sex, profession, status, and so on. The main purpose is to stimulate the formation of groups, alliances, partnership and networks that will generate political power and that can work to improve conditions in the communities.

Communicative planning is a socially interactive process between actors who seek consensus and mutual understanding. This planning practice can mobilize people in a strategic planning process, with the main emphasis on the situation now and in the future, on formulating a vision of the desired future, and strategies for achieving this goal. The process can function as a broad learning process, encouraging personal growth in the entire population of the community. In our opinion, the *transactive planning* model (Friedmann, 1973; 1987; 1992) comes closest to fulfilling this issue. Transactive planning focuses on how people's experience can be used to form policy. The planning is not carried out by experts for the object of the plan, but in face-to-face dialogue between those involved and interested. Personal growth and joint action are the key elements in this planning, and planning is not divorced from other social action in which the aim is to gain control over social processes that affect one's welfare. Transactive planning uses democratic processes to encourage opposition to the established authorities and can, in some situations, result in changes in political power and policy-making. Such mobilization can start with individuals and be expanded to a movement and gain strong political power, and these movements can gradually lose their basis for existence because they have managed to put the issues they are fighting for on the political agenda and made a desired solution part of the production of the established governing system.

Transactive planning emphasizes a broad, grass-roots mobilization to gain the strength to take greater responsibility for one's development and to influence the conditions under which one is working. This planning process transforms knowledge into action through an uninterrupted sequence of relationships between people. Friedmann (1992) argues that knowledge and action can be linked through critical understanding and radical practice, and that the planning process is a far-reaching learning process in which everyone can participate. Friedmann puts it like this: without a vision, there is no radical practice; without radical practice, no formation of a theory; without a theory, no strategy; and without a strategy, no action. These relationships can be illustrated as a learning spiral. After one circuit in the spiral, the actor is back where he/she started, but with new knowledge and in a different situation. The question, then, is whether the new knowledge and understanding of the situation are sufficient reasons to reconsider, one by one, the vision, the strategies, the practice and the theories. In the context of mobilization, this learning spiral will have to operate at several levels. Levin (1988) refers to this as a process where it is usually individuals who go round the first circuit, and they gradually get other individuals, groups and local communities to join them in the spiral of understanding and practice. In the same way, Dryzek (1990) calls this a function of the planning for an *inclusive democracy*, and Sager (1992) talks about integration of people and personal growth.

Strategic planning refers to fundamental questions such as what is typical for the situation with its development characteristics and challenges, what sort of future we want, where we should start, and how we can make changes in order to move from the present situation in the direction of the ideal. Questions such as these touch on ideological values that can be expected to be fairly stable over a period of time. It is, however, a moot point to what degree planning alone can manage to change such standpoints. By strategic factors in local development work, we mean basically that there exists locally a realistic understanding of the present situation and of the future, and that there is a reasonable measure of agreement as to how to act in order to achieve the desired future (vision). Over a period of time, changes will certainly be likely, and therefore strategic planning may be used as a tool to stimulate the acquiring of knowledge, to increase awareness and to bring about a new understanding, in the hope that individuals, organizations and communities can change their behaviour. Formalized collaboration at this planning level can be called *strategic partnerships*. A strategic partnership is reasonably formalized and has a relatively flat hierarchy. The activity is variable, and the number of members is uncertain and changing. These partnerships are often mobilized around a core of members when the situation demands it, and there is a need for a large number of members in order to influence the agenda setting. These partnerships need members that share a common understanding of the situation and a common vision of the future, and have agreed upon strategies. In these partnerships, the partners from the government structure will clearly experience dilemmas when participating in governance structures, because much of the strategic work in governance partnerships is to influence the public sector political agenda.

One important experience from our use of the empowerment planning model is that people easily get mobilized in the discussion of strategic issues that concern them, but, in the political will-formation process, there is a critical stage between the discussion and the actual involvement in organization that can implement actions. Some people seem to be more interested in talking about what others must do than actually taking responsibility for getting something done.

Ethical–political discourses, tactical planning and organization

Ethical–political discourse concerns the conflicts of interest that often are connected with the utilization of resources. These conflicts are right at the core of tactical planning, the aim of which is to obtain and deploy resources among responsible actors. In relation to power dimensions, this involves having the authority to make decisions or, as the case may be, to prevent decisions being taken (Lukes, 1974). Therefore, organization and co-ordination are central themes also in this type of planning, in particular in relation to partnership organizations in regional and local development work, because the implementation of the concrete measures normally must be carried out by the collaborating organizations in the network organization, and not by the partnership itself. In this way, organizing becomes a critical tool in taking the step from mobilization to implementation.

In all regional and local communities, there will be a certain density of organizations and relationships between them. Amin and Thrift (1995) have demonstrated that a high density of organizations is favourable for the communities' relative power and dynamics. It is, for example, a well-known fact that communities dominated by a single enterprise, which thus have a low density of organizations, normally experience great problems when the situation demands readjustment and creativity, because these enterprises have to reduce staff or close down. In other communities, getting people to come forward as entrepreneurs and, if necessary, co-ordinate their efforts can be a big problem. Without a necessary supportive culture that allows room for experimentation and making mistakes, many will find it too much of a burden to come forward as entrepreneurs, whether in the field of business or in other activities.

It is therefore vital to achieve a division of labour and partnership with voluntary associations and organizations, private enterprise, public administration and politicians. It may be an ideal to seek to achieve harmony between local organizations and their surroundings, but, in practice, situations involving conflicts are unavoidable, simply because the organizations must fight for limited resources, split between different and often irreconcilable needs, interests and values.

By organizing, we refer to the fact that empowerment planning through mobilization creates a power that is able to form new organizations and changes in temporary and permanent organizations, and thus to increase the institutional capacity. In this process of organizing, the empowerment process is about using one's own competence, creativity, motivation, raw materials, capital, technology, and so on, in the best possible way to satisfy needs. In addition, empowerment involves looking for partners with whom to co-operate, so that it is possible to complement each other's resources and supplement production, without the development of dependency relationships between the partners.

Ethic–political discourse relates to the questions of organization and co-ordination, which are issues for tactical and co-ordinative planning. Co-ordinative planning sees planning as anticipatory co-ordination. The focus is on how to deploy organizations to undertake the necessary actions, at the appropriate time, to accomplish mutually agreed-upon outcomes. The objective of tactical planning is to develop flexible, short-term planning. This involves giving priority to activities over a period of time in the form of a *programme of action*. The formulation of these programmes can be based on *incremental planning* (Lindblom, 1959; 1979), a form of planning that requires that the people responsible for drawing up the plan of action are in a position of authority (J. Amdam and Veggeland, 1998). Usually, however, these programmes of action can only consider how to use the organization's own resources, such as money and labour. Normally, organizations have scant resources at their disposal and are very dependent on other actors in order to get things done, but programmes of action can stimulate the production of realistic ideas about just what the organizations are in a position to achieve, alone and in *tactical partnerships*.

Tactical partnerships are highly formalized, have a limited number of members, and have a strong need for an agreed-upon and accepted common action programme. In addition, the partners need to get their part of the common action programme prioritized in their own action programmes. As for the strategic partnerships, the partners are caught in a situation of uncertainty. How much can they contribute to the common action programme, and how much involvement are their own organizations willing to accept? If there is a big difference between what the partners say they will do, and what they actually do, they will lose trust and become less important partners in the future.

Lindblom (1959) acknowledges this uncertainty and presents his alternative of disjointed incrementalism as a planning theory that is close to the political reality. Such disjointed planning involves a form of approach in which, by taking small steps forward and adjusting goals and measures, an attempt is made gradually to move forward. Lindblom stresses that this way of creating policies works within the framework of basic values and aims such as full employment and economic growth. It is, therefore, an exaggeration to claim that this small-step planning that Lindblom discusses is without direction. On the other hand, it would appear to be correct to claim that planning, in the main, is a tool in the hands of those with power in the community. Various forms of participatory planning are based on the participation of actors and communication between affected and interested groups.

Advocacy planning (Davidoff, 1973) has as its point of departure that planning must include the population in the democratic process. One way can be that the authorities give poorly organized groups in local communities a spokesperson (an advocate). Advocacy planning can be used to create solidarity and to include poorly organized groups in the process, as done by J. Amdam (1995), who tried to integrate women more strongly in municipality planning. The aim was to make these groups more equal negotiating actors in relation to the authorities, in the process of drawing up and carrying out plans. For this reason, there are obvious similarities between advocacy planning and negotiation planning. Forester (1987; 1993) looks at conflicts and shows that planners, in practice, can be both negotiators and mediators, but that, in addition, they will be expected to be a spokesperson for poorly organized interest. Both forms of planning assume a limited number of actors in order to be operational.

We have learned that lack of responsibility and accountability is a main challenge in the implementation of local and regional action programmes, which normally involve many partners. Therefore, it is very important, when these action programmes are set up, that each collaborating organization takes responsibility for its part of the actions in the programme, and gets its part of the action prioritized in its own organization and action programmes.

Pragmatic discourses, operative planning and implementation

Pragmatic discourse concerns discussion of the facts and data, and is a discourse linked to instrumental rationality and operative planning. From a power perspective, this involves having the knowledge and other resources to implement what has been politically decided, but it also involves preventing the implementation of such decisions (Lukes, 1974). From a communicative perspective, this means having knowledge with argumentative force. In political processes, however, it is often the case that the administration and other experts put forward such knowledge as objective truths and, in that way, stifle political debate. This is particularly unfortunate as much of the relevant knowledge is based on values and is therefore not objective (Morgan and Smircich, 1980). When it comes to the use of knowledge in planning, the challenge is to combine objective truth and argumentative power to form definite alternative courses of action that are appropriate to the situation or the problem one is facing. Flyvbjerg (1993) discusses the rationality of power and puts forward the idea that a project for local planning and development goes through the following phases: genesis, design, decision and implementation. He has found that the most powerful parts of the process are before the design phase and after the decision phase. In this way, the genesis phase and the implementation phase become the most important in the regional and local development process.

By implementation of the actions, we mean the regional or local organizations' possibility to control that the implementation is, as closely as possible, in accordance with visions, strategies, action programmes, and so on. To put it in other words, planning must be an integrated part of the whole policy-making process, not only a limited piece of it. Regional and local organizations need to be empowered with the means to force through what has been democratically decided, and the implementation needs to be supported by the institutional, strategic and tactical planning.

Pragmatic discourse concerns the arguing of facts and data and is a discourse tied to operative planning and instrumental rationality, that is, planning as a deliberative activity of problem-solving, involving rational choices by self-interested individuals or homogenous social units. The objective of rational planning is for the actors to decide to what ends future actions should be undertaken, and what course of action would be most effective. Instrumental rationality, or *synoptical planning*, can be a tool to accomplish these actions, but normally synoptical planning requires an actor who has command power and full control over the implementation (Gunsteren, 1976). Synoptical or rational planning is often presented as an ideal model for planning. This model for planning assumes, among other things, full knowledge about all conditions and distinct, stable goals, and that one is in charge of the means (Banfield, 1973[1959]). From community planning in practice, we know these preconditions can never fully be present. Rational planning is based in instrumental rationality and is strongly connected with the positivists' theory of knowledge. The presumption here is that objective knowledge can be gained through a scientific, hypothetical-deductive process. The controlled experiment stands as the methodical ideal. The founding doctrine for positivism is to achieve control of society through knowledge and technique. The only true views of the world are those that are based on empirical observations. Assertions that are not testable in an analytical or empirical way should be disregarded entirely. This positivist science ideal creates an interest in research aimed at unveiling connections between cause and effect, and establishing power based on causality and evidence.

Operative planning refers to the local capacity or power to implement planned action. This type of planning has as its ideal instrumental and rational planning (Simon, 1965). A prerequisite for this planning is, among other things, that, at the moment of decision, there is full awareness of the present situation and clear and unambiguous objectives for the future, so that it is possible to choose which alternative offers the best course of action. In the context of practical planning, the limited projects come closest to this ideal. However, the preceding institutional, strategic and tactical planning can be seen as an additional aid towards establishing the necessary legitimacy and power of partnerships at the operative level.

Operative partnerships have a very high degree of formalization, mainly externally given legitimacy, a limited number of members, a clear hierarchy and a well-developed specialization, and have a clear focus on getting things done. These partnerships are often organized as projects, and the relationships between the partners are formalized with legally binding contracts based on the previous institutional, strategic and tactical planning. Active involvement from the contract partners is therefore expected, accepted and regulated. Without a contract, it can become impossible to keep partners accountable for action they have agreed to implement when the action is delayed or only partly implemented, or there is no action at all.

With this understanding of planning and partnerships at different levels, we can talk about an *implementation chain*. The operative planning partnerships at one level will be a starting point and a frame for the institutional planning at the level below. In this way, planning at one level can support planning at a lower level with much needed resources, power, acceptance and legitimacy, through institutional partnership agreements (see Figure 3.4). Or, to put it another way, an operative action in a project

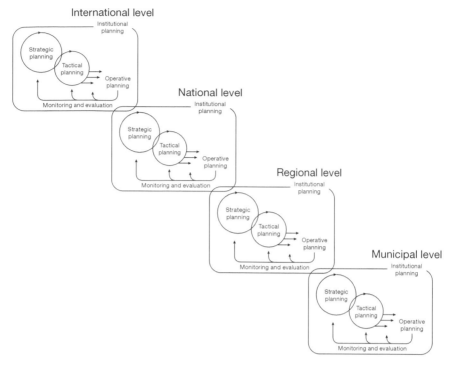

Figure 3.4 The public health chain

at one level can give birth to institutional planning and a new project at a lower level.

Discourses, learning, monitoring and evaluation

In relation to Habermas's model for political will formation, it is unnecessary to include these elements, because they are already, indirectly, parts in the process. However, as regional and local planning and development work is a continual process in which it is important to contribute to the various discourses, we consider monitoring and evaluation as very important opportunities to promote a learning process with all the forms of discourse we have discussed above. Nevertheless, it is essential that the monitoring process, in addition to measuring measurable results, also sets the stage for discourses at the other levels in the planning and development work, that is, institutional, strategic, tactic and operative levels. We have learned, from taking part in regional and local development processes, that monitoring and evaluation must be a democratic process with critical questions, but the process often becomes a cover-up ritual for undone and unsuccessful activities. Accountability is a prerequisite for learning, but there is often a lack of delivered responsibility in the organizations and between the organizations to keep the actors accountable for the outcome. We will discuss monitoring, evaluation and learning in the next chapter.

Conclusions

One of the main observations from studying regional and local planning and development is that the empowerment model outlined above is a sound concept in order to stimulate local, regional and organizational development. However, and in accordance with the theoretical basis for the model, all the variables in the model have to be active if the process is to produce empowerment. Lack of external support and lack of internal mobilization, organization and action can each give an incomplete process. The planning process needs to stimulate all the development variables, particularly those that are the weakest. In addition, we have experienced that the order of stimulating the variables does not matter. To stimulate the weakest variable at any time is always the most successful approach in order to create empowerment.

4 Empowerment evaluation in regional planning and public health work

In the previous chapters, we discussed the governance turn and presented our empowerment-planning model. In these chapters, public health work is regarded as a policy-making process based on governance structures in the form of partnerships between the public, private and voluntary sectors, and between levels of government. Further, the empowerment-planning model is put forward as an appropriate approach to empowerment in local and regional communities, if the planning approach is designed to stimulate the different variables in a development process. In this chapter, we will discuss to what extent the principles of empowerment evaluation can supplement our empowerment-planning model and become a guide in setting up monitoring and evaluation processes, and how the principles can stimulate the learning process in public health work.

Evaluation approaches

There are many definitions of the central terms in evaluation. Evaluation is usually a periodic and episodic exercise, and monitoring is usually a continuous process that provides the evaluation process with data, and signals problems and opportunities that must be addressed. Indicators are collected data and information that demonstrate trends and patterns and that can support the monitoring and evaluation. Evaluations that show high *efficiency* mean optimal use of input (resources) in the production of output. High *effectiveness* means that the production has created desired and meaningful impacts (outcomes).

According to the United Nations (2009: 172), *monitoring* refers to the ongoing collection and analysis of information about trends, activities and events that could influence the plan's performance. Monitoring can also address whether the plan has been efficiently managed through plan administration processes. *Evaluation* tells decision-makers whether, and how effectively, the plan has achieved its intended goals and objectives. Evaluation is the measurement of the plan performance in terms of the outcomes and impacts, compared with the intended goals and objectives, and the efficiency with which related resources have been used and the plan has been administered.

In a comprehensive publication from the WHO, the principles and perspectives on evaluation in health promotion are discussed very thoroughly (WHO, 2001). One of the main conclusions is that evaluation in health promotion is an evolving field, and that one big challenge is to address the issues and problems involved in evaluation. Increased internal and external pressure for evaluation is one of the issues. First, professionals and other internal stakeholders frequently have a strong personal investment in their health promotion intervention. They often want to know whether their efforts have had a positive effect (*outcome* or *impact evaluation*) and the reasons why (*process evaluation*). Second, an increased demand for evaluation of health promotion is rooted in the pressure imposed by governmental and non-governmental funding agencies. They want *evidence of effectiveness*, and particularly cost-related effectiveness (cost-benefit analyses), and evidence that the interventions have been, or are being, implemented as originally intended (WHO, 2001: 521). Not surprisingly, the conclusion after reviewing evaluations of health promotion is a shortage of evidence on effectiveness. This shortage can be explained by several causes. First of all, there is the inherent difficulty of evaluating complex interventions that involve multilevel, multi-sector and multi-strategy interventions that have a poor control over the implementation of health promotion initiatives. A second cause is the lack of accepted appropriate methodologies and methods to collect evidence of effectiveness. Having said that, public health work does not struggle with this problem alone. Reviews of the literature on the effectiveness of initiatives related to nutrition, drug use, physical activity and teenage pregnancy have identified few well-conducted evaluations and consistent findings (WHO, 2001: 522).

This lack of scientific knowledge about the relationships between causes and effects is also a major weakness in *health impact assessment analyses*. These are complicated, highly technical and expert-driven evaluation exercises that very much follow epistemology instrumental rationality. However, the dominance of these analyses is currently being challenged by communicative planning and empowerment approaches (United Nations, 2009: 174).

In the debate on methodology and methods, there are, in theory, two paradigmatical positions (see Chapter 1). One is the traditional, *positivistic and instrumental approach*, which seeks causality between interventions and effects and which inspires people to seek objective knowledge and quantitative evidence of effectiveness. The other is the *phenomenological and communicative approach*, which sees intervention as a capacity-building process and regards subjective and qualitative information from the participants about their interpretation of the situation as valid data. In practice, the main question is how to combine the quantitative and qualitative methods, and, as a consequence, practical evaluation has a mix of methods as a typical characteristic. In addition, public health work is ideologically committed to stimulating empowerment, which, in its nature, must be a balanced blend of instrumental and communicative rationalities, and, therefore, needs to pay attention to the different variables in development processes in addition to the evidence of effectiveness of the process. WHO summarizes its discussion in five conclusions:

1 evaluation should be participatory;
2 evaluation should have adequate resources;
3 evaluation should examine both processes and outcomes;
4 evaluation should use a mix of methodological designs; and
5 evaluation expertise of complex design should be fostered.

(WHO, 2001: 245–55)

These conclusions bring us back to planning. According to the WHO (2001: 524), the process of evaluation is integrally related to the process of planning. Planning and evaluation can be seen as mirror images. Planning, implementation and evaluation are often portrayed as elements of an inter-active cycle: planning leads to implementation, which leads to evaluation, which, in turn, can lead to further development of planning, exactly as we wrote in Chapter 1 about the HEPRO planning circle and in Chapter 3 about empowerment planning.

Learning organizations and regions

Public health work is in its mission cross-sector work and has that in common with regional development work. Indeed, many will say that public health work *is* regional planning and development work. From this point of view, it becomes obvious that public health work is about different organizations collaborating across vertical and horizontal power structures in order to enhance the capacity of the region to handle public health issues. Thus, the monitoring and evaluation process needs to become a process of learning, both in the organizations and in the region.

It can be argued that organizations and regions are sustainable just because they are capable of evaluating and monitoring their actions and, thus, are able to learn from their own actions. Improvement is the key word in evaluation, and learning is the important tool needed in order to achieve the wanted outcomes. Learning can be regarded as a process in which the actors are seeking better ways to realize their interests and values. However, learning is not only about new means to realize individual goals. Learning can also involve changing values, needs and interests at a collective level. That is why it is important to talk about learning as a community development process.

It is often said that individuals learn in a collective interaction process, and that collectives learn through the individuals. However, to some extent, collectives such as organizations and local and regional communities and organizations are independent from the individuals, and collectives develop their own understanding of the situation, goals, strategies, and so on. It is possible to find out what collectives have learned by studying their plans, processes, rules, routines and positions of people in power, how they use power, and so on. This learning is maintained through processes of planning, decision-making and implementation, through socialization and recruiting. Learning thus becomes an important part of local and regional development, and evaluation processes as feedback loops need to be included in the planning system.

In the concept of the *learning organization*, a successful organization needs continually to adapt and learn in order to respond to changes in the environment (both internal and external). The idea of a learning organization is that there is some learning in organizations that takes place over and above the learning undertaken by different individuals as part of their work and experience in organizations. Based on a systemic approach, Senge (1990) identifies and discusses five disciplines that all together create the learning organization. The five disciplines of the learning organization are (1) *personal mastery*, (2) *building shared vision*, (3) *mental models*, (4) *team learning* and (5) *systems thinking*, which is the fifth discipline that integrates the other four. Senge regards learning as a kind of growing, bottom-up process, starting with personal mastery of yourself and then sharing vision with others, reflecting on mental models, bringing in the team and making this become a systematic way of thinking in the organization. Based on this practical understanding of the five-discipline approach to learning organizations, the message from Senge's work can help us to understand why the disciplines to some extent overlap, and how the five disciplines can contribute to individual and collective learning.

In the concept of *learning regions*, knowledge is regarded as the fundamental resource and learning as the most important process (Asheim, 1996). Learning regions are regarded as more competitive in the global economy than traditional industrial districts. The learning region process can make regions more independent of external actors and the importing of knowledge from outside the regions, if the regional learning becomes a public good produced in a collective action process. A region with a great capacity for collective action increases its potential for influencing its environment, but, at the same time, reduces the potential for individual action. Capacity for collective action is thus achieved at the cost of opportunity for individual action. This means that actors must renounce individual advantages to achieve collective goods.

In the concepts of learning organizations and regions, localized knowledge and the process of learning can fundamentally be seen as collective goods. The fundamental question is then which conditions must be fulfilled for these collective goods to be produced in learning organizations and regions. Collective goods can be regarded as non-excludable, which means that a possible user cannot be refused the benefit, even if the user has taken no part in producing the good. This implies that, if one person can utilize the good, every person can utilize it. The opposite of public goods is private goods, which are excludable goods because the producer can sell them to one customer and thus refuse their use to others. If collective goods are to become a meaningful reality, the actors must be able to separate individual interests, needs and values from collective interests, needs and values.

Instrumental action theories such as the rational choice theory explain learning in organizations and regions as collective action from the perspective of rational, self-interested individuals. However, the rational choice theory cannot explain value rational collective actions, such as how to create a social entrepreneur. The *communicative action theory* provides a broader concept that includes different forms of rationality. This theory has a focus on the social learning process between interactive individuals, rather than isolated, self-interested persons. In this way, the theory manages to explain common understanding and collective identity, trust, confidence and other social relations. Communicative processes between persons seem to be a fundamental prerequisite for learning organizations and regions.

Learning at different levels

In addition to understanding learning as an individual and collective process, it is important to talk about learning at different levels. Bateson (1985 [1972]) identifies and discusses learning at four levels, and we have found that these levels can easily be adapted to our empowerment planning model. The four levels are as follows:

- *Learning at level 0* is seen as no learning at all. New situations that seem to be similar to earlier situations are met with the same solution (laws, manuals, legislation and other stable action models).
- *Learning at level I* means choosing among different solutions within a set of options. In a situation with similar information as an earlier situation, the actors are able to choose solutions that are appropriate to the situation.
- *Learning at level II* means the actor is able to choose among sets of options based on different values. Compared with the situation at level I, the actors manage to evaluate and change to another set of value-based alternatives.
- *Learning at level III* is about contextualized level-II learning and is not easily understood, but it may be the existential level meaning setting the framework for learning at different levels, based on learning about how to learn.

These levels correspond to much-used terms in the learning literature such as meta-learning, and triple-, double- and single-loop learning. However, instead of these learning terms, we can use terms from the planning literature: *learning at institutional, strategic, tactical and operative levels.*

Learning at the operative level indicates that rules and old praxis tell us what is to be adequate praxis. This learning is about direct experience, such as: if I put my hand in the fire – it gets burned. In given situations, one runs to the standard solutions to the problems that have been used before (take the hand out of the fire). No other alternatives are regarded as possible solutions. The actors do not know any other way to act. This can be an appropriate action, but it is more likely that the action is dominated by routines, and the action can be a perverse response to the stimuli.

Learning at the tactical level is what we routinely refer to as learning in the form of generalization from basic experiences; for instance, I have experienced 'hand in fire' and 'being burned', and I won't do it again. For this actor, learning is about evaluating action in relation to his/her interests, goals and values. A successful action is an action that reaches the goals he/she has, but these goals are firm and are not changed owing to learning. Action and learning at this level mean that the dominating action pattern gives opportunities to discuss several possible actions, but the goal is the same.

Learning at the strategic level is a kind of change of paradigm, including new values, norms and ends. This learning means: I don't generally risk getting burned, but I might do so to save someone else from a fire. In this situation, the actors not only evaluate the different alternatives to reach the goal, but they evaluate different goals. Learning at the strategic level means that we will be back in learning at tactical and operative levels, but now within a new kind of paradigm. Such learning happens rarely and is a kind of culture revolution that can take place both in organizations and in local and regional communities. In a learning perspective, such a change is to be regarded as in-depth learning. If we want fundamental changes, we need this *deep learning* of new values at the strategic level. Persons and organizations that have learned at this level have internalized new values and adopted corresponding logical courses of action as part of their repertoire of actions. As we know, in public health work, it is now expected that people take more responsibility for their own health, and we say that what we then expect is an example of deep learning. We argue that, if an intervention process such as the HEPRO project does not result in deep learning, then local people most likely will turn back to old habits after the project is ended. Although such higher-level learning undoubtedly takes place, it seems difficult to manage it. To set up a system of learning that stimulates learning at all the levels is a main issue for institutional planning.

Learning at the institutional level appears when the referential framework evolves and the main objectives of the organization or community are modified. Involving organizations in partnership for public health work is an example of institutional changes that create opportunities to develop new systems of learning. The institutional framework and system of learning influence the learning processes at all the other levels and have to be designed very carefully in order to stimulate the wanted learning. In single organizations, the leaders have the overall responsibility to design adequate learning systems. In partnerships and implementation structures such as health promotion programmes, this responsibility is transferred to the leader of the local or regional projects. For all these leaders, the fundamental questions that have to be asked more or less continuously relate to the best ways of stimulating learning at operative, tactical, strategic and institutional levels. At the same time, there is a need to take into consideration that all the levels of learning are interconnected within the system of learning.

Empowerment evaluation and public health programmes

Empowerment evaluation is a rather new concept that is designed to help improve policy programmes. The empowerment concept is based on ten principles, and, in practice, these principles are overlapping and interactively reinforcing (Fetterman, 2005: 27–41):

1 Empowerment evaluations are designed to help people *improve* their programmes. The evaluator's role is to help people to help themselves, and empowerment evaluation is never conducted for the sake of intellectual curiosity alone.
2 The evaluator serves as a coach for the people involved in the programme, or as a critical friend to assist them, ensuring logic, rigour and a systematic approach. However, the *community owns* the evaluation with its conceptual direction and actual implementation.
3 *Inclusion* means inviting as many stakeholders to the table as is reasonable and feasible and encouraging their participation.
4 *Democratic participation* is about how the people will interact and make decisions once they are together. Democratic participation is both a means to ensure equality and fairness, and a tool to bring forth as many insights and suggestions about how to improve the programmes as possible.
5 *Social justice* is a fundamental principle guiding empowerment evaluation in how to treat people, choosing target groups for the programme and selecting data in the evaluation.
6 Local community members have invaluable *knowledge about their community*. If valued, respected and mobilized, this knowledge can be a strong force in improving the community.
7 *Evidence-based strategies*, with a track record and external credibility, allow communities to build their activities on knowledge. However, evidence-based interventions cannot be blindly adopted, but must be adapted to the local conditions and environment.
8 *Capacity building* in empowerment evaluation is about learning how to conduct evaluation and building skills in areas such as evaluation logic, chain of reasoning, logic models, evaluation design, data-collection methods, analysis, reporting and ethics.
9 Capacity building, local and evidence-based knowledge and other principles contribute to the *organizational learning* process. Feedback loops and continual collection of information about staff performance and programme output and outcome are an integrated part of

empowerment evaluation. Conducted in a transparent way, the learning process can ensure that data are credible and used to inform decision-making.

10　Empowerment evaluation is about *accountability*. It is useful for external accountability, but the strength of empowerment evaluation is in fostering internal accountability. External accountability in programme implementation lasts as long as the programme.

Fetterman (2005) argues that there is a dynamic in these ten principles that, in practice, encourages internal accountability. The principles remind people that they are both individually accountable and accountable as a group. Individuals hold one another accountable for promises and commitments, and the feedback mechanisms built into empowerment evaluation hold the programme and the organization accountable. In this process, the role of the *evaluator* becomes crucial, but we find Fetterman's description of the role unclear and complex. Is this an internal or external person? Is this an adviser or an active person in the process? The description of the role seems to indicate a mix, and we will say that there seems to be a special need for discussing and clarifying this role. In addition, the potential conflict between the different roles of the community, funder and evaluator need to be discussed. In practice, they do not have to be in harmony; rather, the normal situation is likely to be that they are in conflict with each other.

In order to understand this critique, we have to turn to the fundamental understanding of empowerment. According to Schulz *et al.* (1995), empowered individuals are critically aware of their situation and therefore able to analyse what must change, possess a sense of control, are capable of acting and engage in participatory behaviours. At the organizational level, empowered groups compete effectively for resources, influence policy and are networked to others.

However, an empirical review of the literature about empowerment evaluation, undertaken by Miller and Campbell (2006: 314), indicates that, although empowerment evaluation advocates the inclusion of the recipients in the programme, they were seldom part of the empowerment evaluation, compared with what one might expect. The goal of empowering citizens who are the beneficiaries of social programmes has become less salient than holding the staff members accountable to the funding institutions. This is a well-known mechanism from implementing policy programmes. The funding agency needs evidence-based knowledge about the output and the short-term outcome from the programme in order to legitimate its role and the use of the money, and this programme logic is always in conflict with making the most deprived groups and communities targets for the programme. This is just an example of how the different roles in the process can be in conflict, and emphasizes the need to clarify the roles.

Miller and Campbell (2006: 314) conclude, in their review of the empowerment evaluation approach, that the concept is not easily distinguished from other approaches to evaluation with the emphasis on participation, collaborative processes and capacity building, and the concept is criticized for not being fully theoretically articulated. In addition, we will say that many of the techniques that are used in the evaluation are the same as, or similar to, those used in empowerment planning and development. It can be argued that empowerment evaluation as a process is very similar to empowerment planning, and that the empowerment evaluation approach can help us to integrate monitoring and evaluation in the empowerment planning approach.

Learning and evaluating in empowerment planning

According to Fetterman (2005), empowerment evaluation can help organizations and communities to learn and to improve their programmes. Empowerment evaluation is conducted with the purpose of improving the programme and should never be conducted for the sake of intellectual curiosity alone. The feedback loops are designed to produce information about how the programme is working (or not working), and to stimulate a discussion about how to make corrective or adaptive changes. As we have seen, in planning today, learning is regarded as an integrated part of planning systems, and learning in empowerment planning and evaluation is a similar and parallel activity. Such planning and evaluation processes need to stimulate learning at the institutional, strategic, tactical and operational levels of the planning.

Evaluation conducted as reporting to superiors has a tendency to hide information that can be used against them, and to report what easily can be quantified. Evaluations that are done in this manner will not allow for sufficient critiquing, and will normally only involve learning at the operative level. This means learning about how the actions and changes were implemented, compared with the programmed action in budgets, action contracts, and so on. Learning that involves changing the objectives at the tactical and strategic levels can be better stimulated in processes that allow actors to participate and thus accomplish increased insight into what the objectives ought to be and how the actions are carried out. Learning at these levels does require that the actors get the opportunity to participate and to monitor the policy-making process, the decision process and the implementation process and to evaluate the products and the impact of the action. Nevertheless, it is essential that the monitoring process, in addition to measuring measurable results, also sets the stage for discourses at the other levels in the planning and development work, that is, institutional, strategic, tactical and operational levels. If we want people in regions and local communities to take part in the development, we need a planning and evaluating process that can promote learning at all levels.

In order to make evaluating and learning an integrated part of the HEPRO project, we asked the partner to report on these questions when we were half-way through the project:

- What have you, as a partner in the HEPRO project, done to create a learning process about public health in your organization and your community/district/county?
- Who in the organization and the community/district/county has learned about public health so far, what have they learned, and how is this learning expressed in the public health work?
- What are the most important outputs and the most significant impacts on the public health situation from the public health project so far?
- What are you planning to do to stimulate the learning process?

Institutional planning – evaluation and learning

In empowerment evaluation, community ownership and democratic participation are core principles and values (Fetterman, 2005), and we will say it is also so in empowerment planning.

Public health programmes such as the HEPRO project are often initiated nationally or internationally and implemented in local communities. A good balance between top-down policy and bottom-up policy is needed if a community is to avoid becoming dependent on external institutions to solve its problems. A public health programme will normally have a local project group (steering group), with representatives from different sectors and levels of government. This is regarded as a starting point for creating ownership, but the local ownership has to be broader and deeper than the project group. Involving people in planning, implementing and evaluation can create ownership, but democratic participation is not the same as inclusion. Whereas inclusion means bringing all the pertinent groups together, democratic participation is about how the groups will interact and make decisions once they are together (Fetterman, 2005: 45). Community ownership and democratic participation can be regarded as an institutional framework for public health work and tools to improve the legitimacy of public health work and, as such, an important part of institutional planning.

Public health institutional planning should have institutional capacity building and enforcing the local power structure as its superior objectives. This involves adding weight to freedom for local and regional communities to be able to make decisions and to practise direct democracy and social learning. This means a struggle where the alliance between civil society and elected representatives fights to make communicative rationality superior to instrumental rationality in their communities. This implies establishing a process of legitimating policies: a process based on undistorted discourses seeking equality of power and a demand for stating reasons in public meetings. The process needs to involve actors from the public, private and voluntary sectors and from local, regional and national levels. Local and regional communities can influence their own development and stand up as political institutions with legitimacy and acceptance if they are able to create a policy legitimating process. Hence, locally based, cross-sector power can become a counterforce and challenge the established vertical power structure in government.

This legitimating process requires a certain integration between system and life world, but not to the extent that they lose their distinctive characteristics. It is rather so that one should find an arena where co-operation is desirable, and where the public sector can provide incentives in order to achieve the development desired in public, private and voluntary sectors. The neglected partner in this kind of planning and development work is civil society, which we can see as a complex culture of ethical values and moral norms shared by most people inside limited local areas. Civil society refers to relationships between people and relationships outside the reach of public government and private enterprises. Research shows that there is still a social power in civil society that can be mobilized and trans-formed into political power, and that the possibility for a functional and territorial, integrated development seems to lie in an alliance between civil society and democratically elected representatives (Friedmann, 1992). They both have power tied up in territories, both can free themselves from the instrumental rationality that is dominating public government and private enterprises, and both can contribute to communicative rationality.

These arguments imply that we in regional and local planning and devel-opment work should concentrate on the planning process as a policy-making and learning process, and on the fact that it is important to have a plan for intervention in the continuous development process. This plan for the inter-vention process should be based upon acknowledgement of the developing variables and of the planning tools that can stimulate these variables (see Chapter 3).

If we choose to organize the intervention as a project, as often done, the superior perspective for the project should be how a process lasting a limited time, the project, can influence the continuous process that development really is. One of the most serious mistakes that can be made is to see the intervention and the project as a process for making planning documents, such as master plans. When this mistake is made, the process is often limited to strategic and tactical planning and not to stimulating the mobil-izing, organizing, action and learning variables.

These are the self-evaluation questions about institutional planning we asked the HEPRO partners to report on when they were half-way through the project:

- What have you, as a partner of the HEPRO project, done to stimulate the legitimacy of the public health work in your organization and your community/district/county?
- How strong is the legitimacy of the public health work in your organ-ization and your community/district/county now?
- What are you planning to do to stimulate the legitimacy?

- What do you think about your role as leader/responsible of the public health project?
- What are the biggest challenges for your public health project now?

Strategic planning – evaluation and learning

Inclusion and social justice are fundamental principles guiding empowerment evaluation, and, in practice, empowerment approaches to public health typically assist people with specific social concerns or injustice. The target groups might include the homeless, battered women, people with disabilities, children or minorities. The principle of social justice keeps the public health work eye on the prize of social justice, equity and fairness. Fetterman put forward a very illustrative example: data from the evaluation might show that a social service programme is not cost-effective, but the social justice agenda might override a decision about eliminating the programme and force the organization to find ways to subsidise the activity (Fetterman, 2005: 47).

Learning at the strategic level means that the actor is able to choose among sets of options based on different values and goals. Compared with the situation at the tactical level, the actor manages to evaluate and change to another set of alternatives. Learning at this level involves a moral dimension (Etzioni, 1988) and can only be achieved through interaction and democratic discourses (Forester, 1993). This process has to be democratically inclusive and concerned with consensus building. This kind of management by arguments (Healey, 1997) is important for mutual learning, but agreements on values and strategies are likely to be incomplete and unstable when it comes to practice, especially if they are not founded in a collective morality.

The stimulation of the mobilizing variable can be done through strategic planning, with the main emphasis on the situation for the local and regional community now and in the future, and on formulating a vision of the desired future. It is also important to formulate the strategies for achieving this goal. The process should function as a broad learning process, encouraging personal growth in the entire population of the region, and it can be similar to the process that transactive planning mentions (Friedmann, 1973). In this way, a local social power can be created that can further be transformed into political power through organization.

Local and regional community members have invaluable knowledge and information about their community. Respecting community knowledge is important in a bottom-up approach to knowledge sharing and development. This knowledge, if mobilized, can be an extraordinary catalyst for change. In empowerment approaches, intervention will always be an arena where bottom-up policy-making meets top-down policy-making, or where community knowledge meets evidence-based knowledge in setting up the *strategic development programmes*. Evidence-based knowledge and strategies have much to offer development programmes: in essence, they offer programme strategies or interventions that have worked in other, similar communities. However, evidence-based strategies cannot and should not be blindly adopted and expected to work in new communities. If combined with community knowledge, they should be considered as useful ideas and models that are potentially adaptable to the local context. Many communities have suffered when interventions have been out of touch with the local environment, culture and conditions (Fetterman, 2005: 48)

These are the self-evaluation questions we asked the HEPRO partners to report on concerning the strategic planning and learning when we were half-way through the project:

* What have you, as a partner of the HEPRO project, done to put public health on the political agenda in your organization and your community/district/county?
* How accepted is public health as an overall goal and guideline for more detailed planning in your organization and your community/district/county now?
* What are you planning to do to mobilize people and put public health more on the political agenda?

Tactical planning – evaluation and learning

Fetterman (2005: 50) writes that the strength of empowerment evaluation is in fostering internal accountability, and empowerment evaluation is used to achieve internal goals and external requirements and outcome. Learning at the tactical level often means choosing among different solutions within a set of options. In a situation with similar information, as in an earlier situation, the actors are able to select solutions that are appropriate to the situation. Taking responsibility is a prerequisite for this learning, but often there is a lack of delivered responsibility in the communities. The overall prerequisite for learning at this level thus becomes to develop partnerships, networks and other forms of co-operation between the actors, and to set up an action programme that distributes responsibility for the implementation. This form of internal accountability is built within the structure of the organization and between partners in the public health action programme when they hold one another accountable for promises, commitments and agreements.

Tactical planning is about creating action programmes that give priority to projects and actions and distribute responsibilities and resources. Tactical planning is about how to use the organization's resources to achieve desired goals. In public health planning, there are several organizations with separate fields of operation, and, in many cases, the actors have to co-operate if they are to succeed in their struggle for an intended development. The establishment of these partnerships requires the actors to share a common understanding of the present and the future. This involves transforming social power into political power by having the people commit themselves to existing and new organizations that can accomplish, through action, the desired operations and changes. We can use *tactical action programmes* as the term for these partnerships and, by this term, understand agreements that regulate the responsibilities between the actors. However, even if the organizations in the partnership clearly know what they want to achieve, and have potential organizations for the implementation of actions, these local and regional organizations normally have limited control of the necessary means. We have learned from development processes that there often is a lack of delivered responsibility in the organizations and between the organizations to keep the leaders accountable for the outcome or lack of outcome. This gives tactical planning a sort of trial and error quality, which is what characterizes incremental planning (Lindblom, 1959).

These are the self-evaluation questions we asked the HEPRO partners to report on concerning the tactical planning and learning when we were half-way through the project:

- What have you, as a partner of the HEPRO project, done to get public health activity decided and organized in your organization and your community/district/county?
- How deeply rooted is public health work in action plans, budgets and daily work in your organization and with your partners in the community/district/county now?
- What are you planning to do to get new public health activities decided and organized?

Operative planning – evaluation and learning

Capacity building is the important aspect of evaluation, but, from an empowerment perspective, the capacity-building process must include more than the capacity to implement programme-defined activities and projects. This broader understanding of the capacity-building process implies that improving the community's total, long-term capacity to implement planned actions is a key issue for empowerment work. If a programme does not increase this capacity, the community might be in a less favourable situation regarding solving its own problems after the programme than before. The community might have become more dependent on external help.

In regional and local planning and development work, the responsibility for actions is normally divided between many organizations and actors in the private, public and voluntary sectors. Therefore, the implementation of actions often requires extensive co-ordination between the actors and an implementing structure. We can use *operative action plans* or *operative partnership contracts* as terms for these structures and, by these, we under-stand agreements that regulate the actors' responsibilities for implementing the actions and changes. Instrumental rationality or synoptic planning can be a tool to accomplish these contracts of action, but, normally, synoptic planning requires an actor who has command power and full control over the implementation. Consequently, negotiation planning between equal actors will normally be the practical way of working in order to accomplish these kinds of contract (see Forester, 1987).

Operative planning is the instrumental way of planning. Healey (1997) calls this form of planning management by performance criteria and output targets. The planners are supposed to have all necessarily knowledge, and actions are secured through command and control. Within the framework of stable action models, the individuals, households, firms and agencies can work out for themselves how to adjust their behaviour. Learning at this level means no learning at all. New situations that seem to be similar to earlier situations are met with the same solution, based on laws, manuals and other stable action models.

Achieving outputs is important in all planning, and these are the self-evaluation questions we asked the HEPRO partners to report on when we were half-way through the project:

• What actions have you implemented in your organization and your community/district/county in order to promote sustainable public health?
• How great is the capacity of the organization and the community/district/county to implement public health actions now?
• What new public health actions/projects are you ready to implement?

Conclusions

The discussion in this chapter shows that planning, implementation, evaluation and learning are linked in a continuous cycle in public health work. Further, the discussion gives arguments to support the view that organizations and regions can become empowered just because they are capable of monitoring and evaluating their actions and are thus able to learn from their own actions. Accordingly, if we want to promote existing and potential learning organizations and regions, there is a need for an approach to planning that manages to combine communicative and instrumental rationality, and to stimulate learning at different levels. The process can contribute to the reviewing and updating of the planning documents, and to the legitimization of public health work, both in organizations and local and regional communities. Such a complete evaluation and learning process must involve the institutional, strategic, tactical and operational levels of planning.

5 Reflections on the HEPRO project

In this chapter, we present a brief introduction to the HEPRO project and the empowerment-planning model that was introduced for the partners in the project, we list the self-reported activities that were implemented and we show how they fit into the empowerment-planning model. The outputs and outcomes that are included in this chapter are from the answers the partners gave to the self-evaluation questions referred to in Chapter 4. This self-monitoring and self-evaluation is an integrated part of the planning model. In our understanding of empowerment, communities will have a better capacity to lead themselves, focus on their challenges, organize themselves and implement actions, and learn from their experiences after the project.

The HEPRO project

The main goal of the HEPRO project was to integrate health considerations into spatial planning and development, and to make an important contribution to a sustainable public health policy in Europe (see Box 5.1). HEPRO consisted of thirty-two partners and brought together people with expert and specialist knowledge and experience from all relevant sectors, across eight countries around the BSR. The project aimed to help share effective ways to promote health and bring the results to the attention of those who need to take action. The project was to carry out a transnational population survey and training programmes and implement concrete findings from the survey in spatial planning processes (Østfold County Council, 2005: 4).

There is no formal evaluation at the end of the project that can clarify to what extent the project has reached its goals. What we can say about the goals for *output* is that the survey of the population's state of health has been successfully completed, and the data have been used across the national boundaries, and a training programme in public health work and local health profiles have been integrated parts of the project. In addition, health profiles and environmental factors related to health have been used as a basis for a public health policy at local and regional levels. When it

Box 5.1 About HEPRO

Along with the rest of Europe, the BSR is facing enormous health challenges. An ageing population, migration of young people from rural areas to the cities, unemployment, an increase in alcohol and drug abuse, mental illness, and lifestyle diseases especially contribute to these challenges.

They require imaginative, complex and diverse solutions. A solution must have its focus not only on risk factors, but also on factors that are positive and promote health conditions for the individuals. We call a broad, inter-sectoral effort like this, 'The New Public Health Effort'.

The HEPRO project was running as a public health project in 2005–8 and was part-financed by the EU in the BSR INTERREG IIIB programme. The national Healthy Cities networks in the BSR were initiative-takers and HEPRO was professionally supported by the WHO. The WHO Healthy Cities approach seeks to put health high on the political and social agendas of cities, and to build a strong movement for public health at the local level. The HEPRO concept is underpinned by the principles of the WHO Health for All strategy and Local Agenda 21.

HEPRO is characterized by:

- a system theoretical approach to policy production;
- a circular and communicative understanding of planning; and
- a spatial and cross-sectoral focus on public health.

HEPRO aimed to integrate health considerations into spatial planning and development.

Strong emphasis was placed on empowerment, including equity, participatory governance and solidarity, inter-sectoral collaboration, and action to address the determinants of health.

Furthermore, the project aimed to make an important contribution to a sustainable public health policy in Europe. The HEPRO planning model is also a part of work with quality development within the public health field.

Among the results from the project are the HEPRO planning model, the HEPRO survey model, a questionnaire that was answered by 33,000 respondents in the BSR, an interactive web page and a database of results for future research purposes. In line with the vision of HEPRO, the project will be followed up by a new project that builds upon, among other things, upon the results and experiences obtained in HEPRO.

We hope that this publication will both inform and inspire towards further work within the HEPRO goal: increased focus on health and well-being in the BSR.

For more information, see www.heproforum.net.

Source: Wangberg and Dyrseth (2008: 5)

comes to the goals for *outcome*, we only have the data collected midway about how the partners evaluated the situation at that time.

When we asked the partners what the most important *outputs* and the most significant *impacts* on the public health situation from the public health project are so far, they answered:

- The HEPRO project has created a background for the development of public health activities through EU support and local projects.
- They were at the starting point, and the most significant impact of the health project so far has been the high level of attention.
- A health centre has been established that should ensure direct contact between the professional environment and citizens with chronic diseases.
- Politicians in the municipality have passed the budget for 2007 with €1.1 million for activities.
- They managed to get health on the political agenda, including a political decision to form a health project committee.
- It is difficult to say what the results of the activities are and what is the result of other social, cultural and economic factors within the family, the neighbourhood, the workplace, etc.
- They expect the most significant outcomes to come from the results of the health survey.

When we sum up the results from a project such as this, it becomes clear that the project has moved the different partners in the direction of fulfilling the goals of the project. However, what the data do not tell us are the great differences between the partners on how they interpreted and implemented the project. There seems to be a systematic difference between the Western and Eastern European partners. Communicative rationality, broad participation and bottom-up policy-making in public health work seem to be far more accepted in the Nordic countries, compared with, for example, Poland. The examples in Boxes 5.2 and 5.3 illustrate fully the differences in the approach to planning, prevention and promotion of public health. In the case of Denmark (Box 5.2), the process is bottom-up oriented and very communicative. In the case of Poland (Box 5.3), the planning is top-down and expert-dominated, and very instrumental in the planning approach. In the Poland case, there seems to be a lack of trust between the experts and the people. We can add that, when the survey data were collected, the survey was sent by mail to and from the respondents in the Western European partners, but had to be collected through personal interviews in the Eastern European countries. Svendsen and Svendsen (2006) compared the social capital in Denmark and Poland, and found a much stronger trust between people and greater trust in the country's political institutions in Denmark than in Poland. We find it plausible that the differences in social capital and trust in the two countries can explain the great differences between the two partners in how they interpreted and implemented the HEPRO project.

Box 5.2 A health policy produced by the citizens of Vejle, Denmark

In Denmark, HEPRO project partner Vejle has successfully managed to involve people in the planning of a new health policy. A combination of several efforts directed at increased citizen participation proved effective. The bottom-up approach was initially inspired by a lecture on empowerment planning held by Professor Roar Amdam at the 2006 HEPRO partner meeting in Lithuania. But why involve the citizens in the planning process? Isn't that what politicians are for? The planners from Vejle came to the conclusion that the policy could not be realized without the active involvement of the citizens. The politicians wished to do so, according to their vision of the community:

- healthy citizens in a healthy municipality;
- equality in health – it should be possible for all citizens to lead a healthy life;
- enjoyment of life as an important factor in health;
- responsibility for your own health; and
- nutrition and exercises.

A change of lifestyle usually demands personal motivation. In addition, involvement from the start gives better results in terms of ownership and responsibility for implementation. The elements in the bottom-up process involved lifestyle cafés, citizens' proposals by e-mail, wall posters in public institutions, health policy questionnaires and the HEPRO survey.

Lifestyle cafes

Six public meetings were held, open to all citizens. The meetings took place in six different towns/districts in the municipality in order to involve citizens from all parts of the municipality. At the meetings, a broad concept of health and health planning was represented:

- there was music on arrival;
- politicians participated in the meetings;
- two citizens representing different stages of life gave their views on healthy living;
- group discussions gave ideas and suggestions for the health policy;
- two stand-up comedians entertained on health issues; and
- there were exercises.

Involvement by e-mail

Citizens of Vejle were invited to write to 'Mrs Nielsen' and express their solutions on how to make the visions become reality. This resulted in fifty e-mails with project plans and ideas, created a lot of public attention, and also made a lot of citizens smile!

Posters

Posters with space for writing placed at schools and other public institutions gave people the opportunity to write down their suggestions for a healthier community. The posters specifically asked for people's opinions and gave insightful advice on what they felt should be done, and how.

These efforts resulted in 1,500 comments and suggestions on health policy issues, which were categorized into different areas or target groups. When forming the new health policy, the politicians of Vejle took all these into consideration. The citizen-created health policy has now been published in a pamphlet.

For more information, see www.vejle.dk/.

Source: Wangberg and Dyrseth (2008: 20–1)

Circular understanding of planning

The HEPRO planning model represents a systematic and comprehensive, long-term approach to public health planning in communities. The aim is to show, step by step, how a plan where health and well-being aspects are highlighted can be carried out and embedded in the ordinary planning in the municipality/county/district. The model is a systematic approach in six steps, linked together in a circle with a dynamic character. The circle follows a planning period of 4 years. The six steps are (Østfold County Council, 2005: 5): attention; insight and new knowledge; building a platform for joint action; implementation; documentation; and evaluation. This last step in the planning circle is an evaluation of structure, process and results, and the evaluation will give input to the starting point for a new planning circle.

When we compared this model with other models used in health promotion planning in Chapter 1, we found many similarities, but many of these models are top-down oriented and based on an instrumental rationality. The HEPRO project is a part of the Healthy City movement, which is characterized by public health work as community development, with a continuous capacity-building process based on broad participation, communication, consensus building, empowerment, partnership, responsibility and community ownership.

In order to get an indication of the HEPRO project as a continuous process, we can look at what the partners answered when we asked them who in the organization and the community/district/county has learned about public health so far, what have they learned, and how is this learning expressed in public health work?

- The politicians in the health committee and the chief of the health department have learned that prevention and health promotion are

Box 5.3 How HEPRO results are used in Poznan, Poland

In Poznan, population health has been integrated into the planning documents of the city for several years. The city's Health Plan for the years 2003–8, as well as the Poznan City Development Plan, 2005–10, both aim at preventive action concerning citizens. The target groups are adults, children, elderly people, disabled people and people with addictions.

However, health measures are not restricted to the health sector. Health considerations have also been integrated into areas such as welfare; improvement of the natural environment; promotion of culture, sports and tourism; safety and order; and development of the infrastructure in Poznan. Outlined below are the recommendations for actions, which are based on the results from the HEPRO survey. The recommendations aim at sustaining the process of preventive health measures in line with the HEPRO planning model.

Population groups important in the planning of city health policy are:

- residents aged 55 years or over;
- residents under 35, in employment; and
- groups showing negative health behaviours.

Table 5.1 Recommendations for action addressed to the general population in Poznan, based on the results of the HEPRO survey

Survey result	Recommended action
60% of residents rate their health status as good	Programmes to maintain or strengthen health
60% said that their health was good enough to undertake any form of activity	Promotion of active lifestyle Programmes to maintain or strengthen health
The most common diseases are back pains, hypertension and disorders in mental health	Promotion of active lifestyle
Almost 30% of residents of Poznan spend their spare time mainly in a passive way	Promotion of active lifestyle
20% of residents feel worn out most of the time	Health actions offering various forms of rest or relaxation
The number of residents who smoke every day is slightly higher than the national average	Programmes motivating residents to give up smoking
Over-consumption of alcohol: 55% believe that reduction of the amount of alcohol consumed is unimportant	Comprehensive programmes that offer an interesting form of relaxation

For more information about the HEPRO survey, see the 'Results' section of www.heproforum.net.

Source: Wangberg and Dyrseth (2008: 27–8)

very important, overriding values, and that a comprehensive effort is necessary.

- Municipal organization public servants and professional groups have learned more about the relationship between physical and social environmental factors, health and well-being.
- In society, there is reason to suggest that knowledge about healthy habits and a health-promoting lifestyle has increased among the municipality's children and youth.

The answers indicate that there has been some learning and that the circular planning process has been understood and adopted, at least by some of the partners. However, we must bear in mind that the partners gave these answers in the middle of the project, and that the situation can be better understood when we look at the answers they gave on the questions linked to the project as a policy-making process.

The system theoretical approach to policy production

In Chapter 1, we argued that health promotion programmes are policy-making, and we discussed how the systemic policy process model could help us to understand the challenges health promotion programmes are facing. This discussion led us to understand health promotion programmes as community development and the building of community capacity and political institutions. This was further analysed and discussed in Chapters 2–4. Our contribution to this discussion is an empowerment planning model where:

1 community capacity processes consist of five variables: context, mobilization, organization, implementation and learning;
2 these variables can be stimulated by planning that consists of institutional, strategic, tactical and operative planning, plus monitoring and evaluation; and
3 Habermas's model of political will formation based on different discourses can contribute to a philosophical and theoretical basis for the model.

Juridical discourse, institutional planning and context

The juridical discourses concern the actual legitimacy and consistency of the rules of law. In our interpretation, they also include the planning documents' normative effect in relation to other plans and to rules of law, norms, regulations and guidelines for governing society. We call this process *institutional planning*. This is a systematic process for developing a frame of reference for future decisions and actions by a region or community. If we compare our understanding of this term with the Laverack and Labonte

(2000) model of community capacity building, the term 'institutional planning' covers what they call leadership, programme management and the role of the outside agent. These elements are important in institutional planning, but we regard institutional planning as a wider term.

We have learned that it is important to emphasize that development can be intensified by way of a project, but that regional and local community development is nonetheless a continuous process. In our advices to the HEPRO project, we therefore said that the project must be understood as an intervention in a continuous public health work process, and therefore the project must carry out activities in co-operation with regional and local partners when they are ready to participate, and not hold back all the activities until action programmes are decided. Often, these actions require partnerships between actors who are able to commit themselves to co-operative networks or formal organizations. We use institutional partnerships as a term for these partnerships, and, by this, we mean judicially binding agreements that regulate the responsibilities between the actors for implementing the measures and changes.

Friedmann (1987) claims that local and regional development cannot be organized and supported by authority bases in society, but has to grow from within local communities. However, planners who come from the outside can, among other things, help to develop a new self-understanding and improve skills in self-help, direct action, negotiating and drawing up effective plans of action to achieve changes in policy processes and structures. Lack of external support and lack of internal mobilization, organization and action can each result in an incomplete process. Regardless of whether the planners are from outside or inside, we argued that monitoring the process is the most important task for the project leader and project management. This argument is in accordance with the theoretical basis for the empowerment-planning model we have outlined in this book. All the variables in the model have to be active if the process is to produce empowerment, and to stimulate the weakest variable at any time is always the most successful approach in order to create empowerment.

Here are some self-reported activities from the HEPRO partners concerning juridical discourses, institutional planning and context:

- collaboration with the HEPRO project, Healthy Cities network, etc.;
- financing of local activities by the National Institute for Health Development;
- structural reform in Denmark that gives an opportunity to build the health sector from the ground up;
- establishing of a steering group, forum for public health, etc., including politicians, health planners and health promoters, and with the health chief represented to follow the process;
- establishing of different political subcommittees to ensure healthy spatial planning;

- a working group on public health and sustainable development work, including, for example, the local district's leading medical doctor, the leader of the child and school health clinic, the co-ordinator for crime prevention, the environmental health expert, the local urban planner and the Local Agenda 21 co-ordinator;
- particular efforts to involve the politicians so that they would have more interest in public health problems;
- collaboration with other organizations and institutions, organized through participation in different networks;
- composition of health plans that cover all areas of politics in the community, for example, utilizing the results from the health survey;
- close involvement of decision-makers, politicians, citizens and different organizations (NGOs, etc.);
- spreading of information on HEPRO project activity and future possibilities, and spreading the information through different channels; and
- networking as a tool to create involvement among citizens.

These activities tell us that being a partner in the HEPRO project has given the local public health work legitimacy, and that the partners use this legitimacy as a platform for cross-sector collaboration, networking, organizing, participation, and so on, in order to get health promotion and ill-health prevention more accepted and legitimized. When we asked them about the challenges they were facing, they answered that the project represents a new organization and that there is a lack of human resources. A common answer is that direct responsibility for public health often went to only one person, the project leader, and often he/she was a co-ordinator of many public health projects. The project leaders reported that they had problems with finding time to prioritize the work and to find proper areas for collaboration. The HEPRO partners reported at that time that the main challenge was to work out health policies with strong involvement of professionals and citizens. They reported a need for increased competence among the different professions, but could already, in the middle of the project, see some increased political and administrative capacity to handle the health promotion work.

Moral discourses, strategic planning and mobilization

The moral discourse concerns norm conflicts and fundamental values. This activity may also be referred to as a consensus-building activity (Healey, 1997; Innes *et al.*, 1994) and may involve developing a broad, common understanding of development features and challenges and visions of what situation one desires, and of strategies for achieving this situation; in other words, agreeing on a political agenda and building up a collective capacity for action. This is at the core of mobilizing and strategic planning.

Strategic planning refers to fundamental questions such as what is typical for the situation with its development characteristics and challenges; what sort of future we want; where we should start; and how we can make changes in order to move from the present situation towards a more ideal situation. If we compare our understanding of this term with the Laverack and Labonte (2000) model of community capacity building, their terms 'participation', 'problem assessment' and 'asking why' are included in our term 'strategic planning'. Formalized collaboration at this planning level can be called strategic partnerships.

One important experience from our action research on strategic planning is that people easily get mobilized in the discussion of strategic issues that concern them, but, in the policy-making process, there is a critical stage between the discussion and the actual involvement in organizations that can implement actions. We argued that a public health survey, as in the HEPRO project, is an important tool in problem assessment of the public health situation in the different regions and districts. A survey gives a lot of different data about how people regard their situation and what impact public health work and other factors have on their situation. However, the data need to be analysed and interpreted if they are to be used in the planning and policy-making process. In addition, there is a need to involve people in the dialogues between the experts and politicians in order to form a common understanding of what problems need to be solved first and how people can contribute to solving the problems. The creation of this common understanding and the mobilization of people and their resources can increase the local and regional capacity to handle the public health problems that are mapped in the survey.

Some self-reported activities from the HEPRO partners on what they have done concerning strategic planning, mobilizing and setting the agenda are as follows:

- use of information and data from the HEPRO survey for the formation of public heath strategy/health promotion and ill-health prevention plan and other activities;
- information given to politicians, decision-makers and general population about health status of the municipality;
- theme days regarding the result of the health profile, together with the local forum, the political dialogue committee, political subcommittees, project committees and the administrative organization, voluntary societies and the collaboration partners on the health areas;
- getting the politicians involved and placing the health projects on the political agenda, establishing a health prize and campaigns, for example press campaigns;
- keeping health issues on the politicians' agenda through initiation of a number of activities, most of them based upon citizen involvement strategies;

- site visits, study trips and meetings regarding health promotion and ill-health prevention in the HEPRO context, where politicians and the decision-makers participated;
- a campaign to promote citizen involvement in the realization of a municipal health policy; and
- relating people to planning and plan documents via communications and dialogue, for example, contact via municipal services (the strategy has been to educate public servants and reward relevant efforts), contact with the voluntary charitable organizations (the strategy has been economic and practical support of activities), and public participation in municipal planning.

From the answers, we can read that the empowerment planning approach is understood and used. Broad participation is reported to be an important tool in problem assessment and interpretation, and a main goal for strategic planning is to put health promotion on the political agenda and to include health promotion activities in the planning documents.

Ethical–political discourses, tactical planning and organization

Ethical–political discourse concerns the conflicts of interest that often are connected with the utilization of resources. These conflicts are right at the core of tactical planning, the aim of which is to obtain and deploy resources among responsible actors. This involves having the authority to make decisions, or, as the case may be, to prevent decisions being taken. Therefore, organization and co-ordination are central themes in public health work, because the implementation of the concrete measures normally must be carried out by the collaborating organizations in partnerships, and not by the partnership itself. In this way, organization becomes a critical tool in taking the step from mobilization to implementation. By organization, we refer to the partnerships between voluntary associations and organizations, private enterprise, public administration and politicians. If we compare our understanding of tactical planning with the Laverack and Labonte (2000) model of community capacity building, the term 'tactical planning' includes what they call resource mobilization, links with others and organizational structures.

The objective of tactical planning is to develop flexible, short-term planning and to give priority to activities over a period of time. Tactical planning is about making action programmes, allocating budget resources, setting up cross-sectoral working groups, involving the private and voluntary sectors in community development projects, and so on. Usually, however, these programmes of action can only consider how to use the organization's own resources, such as money and labour, but programmes of action can stimulate the production of realistic ideas about just what the local organizations are in a position to achieve, alone and in tactical partnerships.

We have learned that lack of responsibility and accountability is a main challenge in local and regional action programmes. Therefore, it is very important, when local and regional action programme are set up, that each collaborating organization takes responsibility for its part of the actions in the programme, and gets that part prioritized in their own organizations and action programmes.

We have experienced that tactical planning often becomes a battlefield between the power of vision and expectations and the power of resources and realism, and the outcome of the battle is normally compromises linked together in an incremental process, where only small changes of direction can be obtained. However, small changes in the right direction can, over time, add up to big changes. So, in our advices to the HEPRO project, we said that, in addition to organizing for the big changes, it is important to have a clear focus on the small changes and create a lasting platform for common actions.

Some self-reported activities from the HEPRO partners concerning tactical planning, organizing and decision-making are as follows:

- development of a political and administrative structure concerning promotion of health issues and preventive issues, which will be the carrying capacity in regards to solving present and future assignments;
- close co-operation with the public health service suppliers;
- deeper and more active co-operation of public health sector and municipality administration and council;
- involvement of politicians and representatives of municipality administration in public health discussions;
- health impact assessment (HIA) used as a tool when making political decisions;
- assessment of health and environmental consequences of all proposals, in physical planning and in political decisions;
- a check list to ensure that public health is a focus in all planning;
- environmental management system (ISO 14001) – community worked for certification in 2007;
- working on a plan for the environment that also includes a health focus;
- new public health measures adopted as part of the activity and economy plans for the coming year and budgets;
- public health initiatives given priority and funded as part of the annual plans;
- creation of organizations and centres of preventive activities;
- projects organized in collaboration with voluntary charity organizations and/or the county; and
- NGOs encouraged to carry out public health initiatives and organize activities.

According to these activities, the HEPRO partners have been mobilizing resources, networking, organizing, planning and integrating public health perspectives in their daily work. At this stage in the project, it was a little unclear to what extent these activities clarified the responsibility between the different actors or partners, and to what extent they were accountable for their part of the mutual activities. However, Box 5.4 shows how Sønderborg in Denmark has integrated health impact assessment into the municipality decision-making process.

Pragmatic discourses, operative planning and implementation

Pragmatic discourse concerns discussion of the facts and data, and is a discourse linked to instrumental rationality and operative planning. From a power perspective, this involves having the knowledge and other resources to implement what has been politically decided, but it also involves preventing the implementation of such decisions. Operative planning refers to the local and regional capacity or power to implement planned action, and the preceding institutional, strategic and tactical planning can be seen as an additional aid towards establishing the necessary political power to implement actions at the operative level.

In Chapter 1, on institutional, strategic and tactical planning, we compared our model with the Laverack and Labonte (2000) model, with nine capacity-building domains, but their model has no domain called the capacity to act. We say that this is a common weakness with all models that are based on instrumental rationality. They tend to under-communicate the problems of having the power to get plans and decisions put into action. The understanding is that knowledge gives experts and politicians power, and that power can be used to implement actions. Often, in development processes, the problem is not to make the decision, but to get the decision implemented.

As we have written earlier in this book, the main goal of health promotion is to empower people to take more responsibility for their own health, but, in order to take on that responsibility, they need increased capacity to act. In empowerment-based public health work, it is you and I, as ordinary people, who are expected to implement new actions. A basic motivation for action is 'what is in it for me?', but, in addition, a successful process needs enthusiasts with the knowledge, competence, capacity, creativity and time to engage in activities to the benefit of society and the common good.

Some self-reported activities from the HEPRO partners concerning operative planning, implementation and actions are as follows:

- different kinds of plans/strategies have been implemented where public health is included;
- education of the employees of the municipality in collaboration with local educational institutes;
- activities for employees: 'training creates well-being' and a 'training group to prevent sickness';

Box 5.4 Development of a health impact assessment tool in Sønderborg, Denmark

It is commonly accepted that sectors outside the health sector have significant impact on the population's health status. Activities in the housing, environment, labour, traffic and social sectors are among the most important determinants for the health status of the population, which is why it is essential to work with an HIA in relation to activities within these sectors.

On the basis of this, the Division for Health in Sønderborg has developed a screening tool to be used in other divisions to determine if, and to what extent, an HIA must be carried out. The screening tool is compiled on the basis of a simple model with three questions, originally used in Nordborg municipality. The model was further developed for an institutional application in Sønderborg municipality. The screening form is completed as indicated in the form. Subsequently, the screening form will state that an HIA screening has been performed, and that the assessment is one of the following:

1   It is determined that the proposal is without significant health impact on the population and/or particular groups in the population.
2   It is determined that the proposal requires a short statement of the health impacts on the population or particular groups in the population.
3   It is determined that the proposal requires a health impact assessment.

Concerning number 1, no further actions will be carried out. Concerning number 2, a short account will be drawn up, starting with the influences and health impact noted in the screening form. The focus is on both positive and negative consequences. It is possible to use the listed guidelines. Concerning number 3, a health impact assessment will be carried out, using the listed guidelines.

Subsequently, the screening form is mailed to the Division of Health. This enables the Division of Health to perform continuous assessments of the practical use of the screening tool. The model is evaluated twice a year.

The screening tool is constructed so that each question is assigned a value. On all indicators, short-term consequences have the same value – therefore, they have the same outcome in the screening tool. The screening tool is constructed so that, if at least one of the questions has short-term consequences, the conclusion will be that the proposal requires a short statement of the health impact.

In relation to long-term consequences, there is a differentiation between positive and negative consequences in the screening tool.

It has no significance for the outcome of the screening whether the consequences are relevant to a particular group or the entire population. This statement is helping in the eventual further analysis. The creation of an HIA builds on the screening performed. The HIA begins by highlighting the indicators that have been marked as having an impact on the health status in the screening form.

The HIA tool and guidelines are available from www.heproforum.net, under 'Results' and 'Planning tools'.

For more information about Sønderborg, see www.sonderborg.dk.

Source: Wangberg and Dyrseth (2008: 25)

- in collaboration with a college, public health servants have been offered courses in health promotion;
- training programmes/education and seminars about public health for local municipality employees, employees of own organization, school nurses, family doctors and public in general;
- forums for citizens to participate in and get involved, stimulation to participation in community development (children and youths are especially prioritized);
- health-promoting regional centre works with schools and youth;
- health centre realized seminars for school nurses, family doctors, etc.;
- actions aimed at vulnerable groups and individuals – youth health centres, guidance groups for parents and pregnant women, facilitated physical training for the elderly, integration of handicapped people, programme for alcoholism and drug abuse;
- welfare department has co-operation with NGO 'Youth federation', to provide social work on streets of the city;
- day centre for persons with mental disabilities;
- development of sports, outdoor activity, walking and bicycling possibilities and activities;
- social meeting places to prevent isolation and loneliness;
- support of, and collaboration with, voluntary charity organizations; and
- no smoking in all public workplaces from 1 January 2007.

The implemented activities that are listed above show that there are a lot of activities that can contribute to personal and local empowerment and capacity building, and these activities indicate that the overall goal of the project, empowerment and personal and collective capacity building, is accepted and implemented.

Discourses, learning, monitoring and evaluation

In relation to Habermas's model for political will formation, it is unnecessary to include these elements, because they are already indirectly part of the process. However, as local and regional planning and development work is a continuous process in which it is important to contribute to the various discourses, we consider monitoring and evaluation as very important opportunities to promote a learning process with all the forms of discourse we have presented above.

Learning at the operative level indicates that rules and old praxis tell us what is to be adequate praxis. In given situations, one turns to the standard solutions to problems that have been used before. No other alternatives are regarded as possible solutions. The actors do not know any other way to act. This can be an appropriate action, but it is more likely that action is dominated by routines, and the action must be regarded as a perverse response to the stimuli.

Learning at the tactical level is based on the rational, goal-oriented actor. For this actor, learning is about evaluating action in relation to his interest, goals and values. A successful action is an action that achieves the goals he has, but these goals are firm and are not changed because of learning. Action and learning at this level mean that the dominating action pattern gives opportunities to discuss several possible actions, but the goal is the same.

Learning at the strategic level is a kind of change of paradigm, including new values, norms and ends. In this situation, the actors not only evaluate the different alternatives to achieve the goal, but they evaluate different gaols. Planning in this situation means a process of both making sense and making action. Learning at the strategic level means that we will be back at learning at tactical and operative levels, but now within a new kind of paradigm. Such learning happens rarely and is a kind of deep learning of new values. If we want people in local communities to take part in development, we need a planning and monitoring process that can promote learning at all levels. To set up this system of meta-learning is the main issue for planning and *learning at the institutional level*.

To collect data about the process and the output is normally an easy part of this monitoring process. However, to obtain data about the outcomes and impacts and then establish plausible causality between the input from the public health work and the impact on the public health work are far more demanding and complicated. Therefore, there seems, in projects such as the HEPRO project, to be a bias towards reporting the easily collected data about the output and neglecting the more difficult data about the outcomes. This lack of data has consequences for the learning process, because there is a need for data about the impacts of the intervention in order to legitimate the public health work, keep it on the political agenda, involve more people and enforce the capacity to handle public health issues.

We have learned from experience in local and regional development work that reporting must be a transparent, communicative and democratic process with critical questions, but the process often becomes a cover-up ritual for undone and unsuccessful activities. Accountability is a prerequisite for learning, but there is often a lack of delivered responsibility in the organizations and between the organizations to keep the leaders accountable for the outcome.

Some self-reported activities from the HEPRO partners concerning reporting, monitoring and learning are as follows:

- meetings, talks, discussions, reflections about health, personal and professional values;
- concept clarification of the broad health and environment concept in the physical planning;
- education in the public schools;
- results and experiences summarized through predetermined evaluation reports;

- environmental certification to stimulate learning through regular evaluations;
- co-operation with state agency health-promoting centre, taking part in their public activities, giving customers free places for activity-realizing and, in everyday work, using materials from the centre – booklets, posters, etc.;
- dissemination of public health information though news papers and Internet;
- carrying out different training programmes, site visits between partners, also exchanging experts in public health and other health-related matters;
- involving citizens in development and implementation of the policy on health;
- networking: cross-sectoral and multidisciplinary co-operation – such as health care professionals, planners, social advisers, economists; and
- encouraging organizations to create public health projects.

Many of these activities are outputs and outcomes that can contribute to learning at the tactical and operative levels, but the outputs and outcomes on strategic and institutional planning are more diffuse. One of the main questions that have to be raised in that respect is to what extent the project has improved the HEPRO partners' capacity to handle health promotion and ill-health-prevention issues, and to what extent the process has contributed to the empowerment of individuals and communities. We will discuss these questions and try to conclude in the following sections.

The spatial and cross-sectoral focus on public health

The HEPRO project's planning approach has strong emphasis on empowerment, including equity, participatory governance and solidarity, intersectoral collaboration, and action to address the determinants of health. Empowerment implies a gathering of power in a dynamic way over a period of time. One method of empowerment is to transfer power from the top down, involving an empowerer and those empowered. Another way is where power is created from the bottom up, by somebody who previously perceived him- or herself to be powerless. Like Laverack and Labonte (2000), we understand the health promotion approach as a combination of top-down and bottom-up policy-making, but there is no single answer on how this balance should be; rather, it needs to be sorted out in the actual situation and context. The implication of this understanding of empowerment is that, after the project, the partners will have a better capacity to lead themselves, to focus their challenges, organize themselves, implement actions and learn from their experiences. In this way, public health planning becomes a broad social learning and mobilization activity that is supposed to enhance the individual and collective capacity in local and regional communities to take care of public health.

From our point of view, the main question in the HEPRO project is how to empower individuals, organizations and communities so they can contribute to a sustainable public health policy. In order to achieve this, it can be fruitful to regard the project as a cross-sectoral and cross-level policy-making and institution-building process.

Regional territorial and horizontal power is weak compared with sectoral and vertical power in most Western countries' political power structures. The first is mainly a part of a territorial, bottom-up regime of governance partnership, mobilization and competition between regions. The second is mainly a part of a top-down regime dominated by government structure, sector thinking, central planning and control of the welfare state production. It can be argued that the situation in general is a consequence of the modernization process in our societies (see Giddens, 1997). In this process, instrumental rationality and top-down policy seem to dominate over communicative rationality and bottom-up policy. Modern societies suffer under instrumental rationalities and the neglect of communicative rationalities and collective processes. Habermas (1995), Friedmann (1992) and others argue that the solution to the problem is to mobilize territorial power to meet sectoral power in a political process. In a regional and local policy context, this means that the bottom-up, mainly communicative power can be used to equalize the top-down, mainly instrumental power and to build adequate regional and local development institutions.

However, in practice, top-down and bottom-up policy-making seems to become more separated than integrated, and the new governance structure seems to exist in the shadow of the old governance structure. In fact, local and regional planning and development work more and more seem to take the form of a two-parallel system: (1) government-dominated, highly sectorized and single-organization planning and (2) governance-based, territorial or spatial planning that tries to foster collaboration and partnership (R. Amdam, 2004). As far as we can draw conclusions from our discussion in this book, there seems to be a similar governance turn in public health work, and the experiences from this turn seem to be similar to the experiences from regional policy.

In order to make a territorial counterforce to the sectorized power that dominates modern societies, partnerships in public health as well as local and regional development need to create legitimacy from inside the community and achieve legitimacy from outside. But this is a kind of dilemma. Partnerships within the governance structure need to be strong enough to influence their partners from the government structure, but is that possible in governance-based partnerships, where the participants from the government structure are free to leave? There is, in local and regional planning and public health work, a great need for empowerment planning as a capacity- and institution-building process that integrates top-down and bottom-up policy-making. There is no fixed balance between top-down and bottom-up policy-making.

Some last words about trust

One of the main observations we have from the HEPRO project, and from other local and regional planning and development projects, is that the empowerment planning model outlined above is a sound concept to stimulate local, regional and organizational development. However, the empowerment-planning model must be implemented with respect for the situation and context, and trust is one key factor that differs from place to place. Trust between politicians, experts and people is the foundation for participation and community capacity building. It takes time to build trust between people, and it can easily be destroyed. Lack of trust can be used as an argument for executing top-down policy with little participation, but, without participation, there is no increased trust. When we look at output and outcome from the process, there are great differences between the partners, and, to a large extent, the differences can be explained by how, and under which conditions, the process was implemented.

Appendix
List of HEPRO partners

Norway

Partner 1	Østfold County Council
Partner 2	Norwegian National WHO Healthy Cities Network
Partner 3	Oppegaard Municipality
Partner 4	Søndre Nordstrand Municipality
Partner 5	Vestvaagøy Municipality
Partner 6	Nordland County Council
Partner 7	Brønnøy Municipality
Partner 8	Odda Municipality
Partner 9	Sandnes Municipality
Partner 10	Kristiansand Municipality
Partner 11	Spydeberg Municipality
Partner 12	Vaaler Municipality
Partner 13	Melhus Municipality

Denmark

Partner 14	Danish National WHO Healthy Cities Network
Partner 15	Danish National Institute of Public Health
Partner 16	Norborg Municipality
Partner 17	County of North Jutland
Partner 18	Vejle Municipality
Partner 19	Holbæk Municipality

Poland

Partner 20	Polish National WHO Healthy Cities Association
Partner 21	Lodz City
Partner 22	Warsaw Municipality
Partner 23	Poddebice Municipality
Partner 24	Poznan Municipality
Partner 25	Olsztyn Municipality

Latvia

Partner 26	Cecis District Council
Partner 27	Saldus District Council
Partner 28	Jurmala City

Lithuania

Partner 29　　Alytus City

Estonia

Partner 30　　National Institute for Health Development

Finland

Partner 31　　Baltic Region WHO Healthy Cities Association

Sweden

Partner 32　　Lund University

References

Amdam, J. (1995) 'Mobilization, participation and partnership building in local development planning: experience from local planning on women's conditions in six Norwegian communes', *European Planning Studies*, 3(3): 305–32.

Amdam, J. and Amdam, R. (2000) *Kommunikativ planlegging*. Oslo: Samlaget.

Amdam, J. and Veggeland, N. (1998) *Teorier om samfunnsplanlegging. Lokalt, regionalt, nasjonalt, internasjonalt*. Oslo: Universitetsforlaget.

Amdam, R. (1997a) *Den forankra planen. Drøfting av kriterium for alternativ næringsplanlegging*. Forskingsrapport 25. Volda: Volda University College and Moere Research Volda.

Amdam, R. (1997b) *Den forsømde regionen. Evaluering av næringsplanlegginga i Ålesund-regionen*. Forskingsrapport 26. Volda: Volda University College and Moere Research Volda.

Amdam, R. (1997c) 'Empowerment planning in local communities', *International Planning Studies*, 2(3): 329–45.

Amdam, R. (2001) 'Empowering new regional political institutions – a Norwegian case', *Journal of Planning Theory & Practice*, 2(2): 169–85.

Amdam, R. (2002) 'Sectorial versus territorial regional planning and development in Norway', *Journal of European Planning Studies*, 10(1): 99–112.

Amdam, R. (2004) 'Spatial county planning as a regional legitimating process', *European Journal of Spatial Development*, ISSN 1650–9544, Refereed article, September (11).

Amdam, R. (2005) *Planlegging som handling*. Oslo: Universitetsforlaget.

Amin, A. (1999) 'An introductional perspective on regional economic development', *International Journal for Urban and Regional Research*, 23(2): 365–78.

Amin, A. and Thrift, N. (1995) 'Globalization, institutional "thickness" and the local economy', in P. Healey *et al.*, *Managing cities: the urban context*. London: John Wiley & Sons.

Arnstein, S. R. (1969) 'A ladder of citizen participation', *Journal of the American Institute of Planners*, 35(4): 216–24.

Asheim, B. T. (1996) 'Industrial districts as "learning regions": a condition for prosperity', *European Planning Studies*, 4(4): 379–400.

Asthana, S., Richardson, S. and Halliday, J. (2002) 'Partnership working in public policy provision. A framework of evaluation', *Social policy and administration*, 36(7): 780–95.

Baldersheim, H. (2000) *Fylkeskommunen som utviklingsaktør: Handlingsrom og legitimitet*. Forskingsrapport 1/2000. Det samfunnsvitenskapelige fakultet. Oslo: University of Oslo.

Banfield, E. C. (1973[1959]) 'Ends and means in planning', in A. Faludi (ed.) *A reader in planning theory*. Oxford: Pergamon Press.

Barton, H. and Tsourou, C. (2000) *Healthy urban planning. A WHO guide to planning for people*. London, New York: The Spon Press.

Bateson, G. (1985[1972]) *Steps to an ecology of mind*. New York: Ballantine Books.

Bennett, R. J. and McCoshan, A. (1993) *Enterprise and human resource development. Local capacity building*. London: Paul Chapman Publishing.

Böhme, K. (2002) *Nordic echoes of European spatial planning*. Nordregio R2002: 8. Stockholm: Nordic Centre for Spatial Development.

Bolan, R. S. (1980) 'The practitioner as theorist. The phenomenology of the professional episode', *Journal of the American Planning Association*, 46(3): 261–74.

Bryson, J. N. and Roering, W. D. (1987) 'Applying private-sector strategic planning in the public sector', *Journal of the American Planning Association*, 53(1): 9–22.

Bukve, O. and Amdam, R. (2004a) 'Regionalpolitisk regimeendring og regional utvikling', in R. Amdam and O. Bukve (eds) *Det regionalpolitiske regimeskiftet – tilfelle Norge*. Trondheim: Tapir akademisk forlag.

Bukve, O. and Amdam, R. (2004b) 'Regimeskifte på norsk', in R. Amdam and O. Bukve (eds) Det *regionalpolitiske regimeskiftet – tilfelle Norge*. Trondheim: Tapir akademisk forlag.

Christensen, T. and Lægreid, P. (2002) *Reformer og lederskap. Omstilling i den utøvende makt*. Oslo: Universitetsforlaget.

Christensen, T. and Lægreid, P. (2003) 'Transforming governance in the new millennium', in T. Christensen and P. Lægreid (eds) *New public management. The transforming of ideas and practice*. Aldershot: Ashgate.

Christensen, T. and Lægreid, P. (2004) *The fragmented state – the challenges of combining efficiency, institutional norms and democracy*. Working paper 3. Bergen: Stein Rokkan Centre for Social Studies.

Corso, L. C., Wiesner, P. J. and Lenihan, P. (2005) 'Developing the MAPP community health improvement tool', *Public health management practice*, 11(5): 387–92.

Davidoff, P. (1973) 'Advocacy and pluralism in planning behaviour', in A. Faludi (ed.) *A reader in planning theory*. Oxford: Pergamon Press.

Dryzek, J. S. (1990) *Discursive democracy. Politics, policy, and political science*. Cambridge: Cambridge University Press.

Dunford, M. F. (1994) 'Winners and losers: the new map of economic inequality in the European Union', *European Urban and Regional Studies*, 1(2): 95–114.

Easton, D. (1965) *A system analysis of political life*. New York: Wiley.

Eriksen, E. O. (1993) *Den offentlige dimensjonen*. Verdier og styring i offentlig sektor. Tromsø/Bergen: Tano.

Eriksen, E. O. (1994) *Politikk og offentlighet. En introduksjon til Jürgen Habermas' politiske teori*. LOS-senter Notat 9405. Bergen: Norsk senter for forskning i ledelse, organisasjon og styring.

Etzioni, A. (1988) *The moral dimension. Toward a new economics*. London, New York: The Free Press.

European Community (1997) *The EU compendium of spatial planning systems and policies*. Luxembourg: Office of Official Publications of the European Community.

European Community (1999) *ESDP European spatial development perspective*. Luxembourg: Office of Official Publications of the European Community.

Faludi, A. (2006) 'The European spatial development perspective shaping the agenda', *European Journal of Spatial Development*, ISSN 1650–9544, Refereed articles November (21).

Fetterman, D. M. (2005) 'Empowerment evaluation principles in practice', in D. M. Fetterman and A. Wandersman (eds) *Empowerment evaluation principles in practice*. New York: Guilford.

Flyvbjerg, B. (1993) *Rationalitet og Magt*. Bind 1 and bind 2. Odense: Akademisk Forlag.

Flyvbjerg, B. (1996) 'The dark side of planning: "rationality and realrationalitat"', in S. J. Mandelbaum *et al.* (eds) *Explorations in planning theory*. Rutgers: Centre for Urban Policy Research.

Forester, J. (1987) 'Planning in the face of conflict: negotiation and meditation strategies in local land use regulation', *Journal of the American Planning Association*, Summer: 303–14.

Forester, J. (1993) *Critical theory, public policy and planning practice: toward a critical pragmatism*. Albany, NY: University of New York Press.

Friedmann, J. (1973) *Retracing America. A theory of transactive planning*. Garden City, NY: Anchor Press/Doubleday.

Friedmann, J. (1978) 'Epistemology of social practice: a critique of objective knowledge', *Theory and Society*, 6: 75–92.

Friedmann, J. (1987) *Planning in the public domain. From knowledge to action*. Princeton, NJ: Princeton.

Friedmann, J. (1992) *Empowerment. The politics of alternative development*. Cambridge, MA, Oxford, UK: Blackwell Publishers.

Friedmann, J. and Weaver, C. (1979) *Territory and function. The evolution of regional planning*. London: Edward Arnold.

Giddens, A. (1984) *The constitution of society*. Cambridge: Polity Press.

Giddens, A. (1997) *Modernitetens konsekvenser*. Oslo: Pax Forlag.

Gillies, P. (1998) 'Effectiveness of alliances and partnerships in health promotion', *Health Promotion International*, 13(2): 99–120.

Green, L. W. and Kreuter, M. W. (2005) *Health program planning. An educational and ecological approach*. London: McGraw-Hill.

Gunsteren, H. R. van (1976) *The quest of control. A critique of the rational-central-rule approach in public affairs*. London: John Wiley & Sons.

Habermas, J. (1984) *The theory of communicative action. Volume 1: Reason and the rationalization of society*. London: Heinemann.

Habermas, J. (1987) *The theory of communicative action. Volume 2: Lifeworld and system: a critique of functionalist reason*. Boston, MA: Beacon Press.

Habermas, J. (1992) *Faktizität und Geltung*. Frankfurt: Surhkamp.

Habermas, J. (1995) *Between facts and norms: contributions to a discourse theory of law and democracy*. Cambridge: Polity Press.

Haines, A., Kuruvilla, S. and Borchert, M. (2004) 'Bridging the implementation gap between knowledge and action for health', *Bulletin of the World Health Organization*, October, 82(10): 724–33.

Hajer, M. and Zonneveld, W. (2000) 'Spatial planning in the network society – rethinking the principles of planning in the Netherlands', *European Planning Studies*, 8(3): 337–55.

Healey, P. (1993) 'Planning through debate: the communicative turn in planning theory', in F. Fischer and J. Forester (eds) *The argumentative turn in policy analysis and planning*. Durham, London: Duke University Press.

Healey, P. (1997) *Collaborative planning. Shaping places in fragmented societies.* London: Macmillan Press.

Healey, P. (1999) *Institutional capacity-building, urban planning and urban regenerating projects.* Paper presented at the XII AESOP Congress. Aveiro: University of Aveiro.

Healey, P. (2001) *Spatial planning as mediator for regional governance.* Paper for the EuroConference on Regional Governance: new modes of self-government in the European Community. Hanover, 19–21 April.

HEN (2006) *What is the evidence on effectiveness of empowerment to improve health?* Health evidence network, World Health Organization, Europe. Copenhagen: WHO regional office for Europe.

Hood, C. (1991) 'A public management for all seasons?', *Public Administration*, 69(Spring): 3–19.

Huang, C.-L. and Wang, H.-H. (2005) 'Community health development: what is it?', *International Nursing Review*, 52: 13–17.

Hyung Hur, M. (2006) 'Empowerment in terms of theoretical perspectives: exploring a typology of the process and components across disciplines', *Journal of Community Psychology*, 34(5): 523–40.

Innes, J., Gruber, J., Thompson, R. and Neuman, M. (1994) *Co-ordinating growth and environmental management through consensus-building.* Report to the California policy seminar. Berkeley, CA: University of California.

Jacobsen, K. D. (1964) *Teknisk hjelp og politisk struktur.* Oslo: Universitetsforlaget.

Jacobsson, K. (1997) 'Discursive will formation and the question of legitimacy in European politics', *Scandinavian Political Studies*, 20(1): 69–90.

Jessop, B. (1997) 'A neo-Gramscian approach to the regulation of urban regimes: accumulation strategies, hegemonic projects, and governance', in M. Lauria (ed.) *Reconstructing regime theory: regulating urban politics in a global economy.* London: Sage.

Keating, M. (1996) *The invention of regions. Political restructuring and territorial government in western Europe.* Oslo: Norwegian Nobel Institute.

Labonte, R. and Laverack, G. (2001a) 'Capacity building in health promotion, part 1: For whom? And for what purpose?' *Critical Public Health*, 11(2): 111–27.

Labonte, R. and Laverack, G. (2001b) 'Capacity building in health promotion, part 2: Whose use? And with what measurement?', *Critical Public Health*, 11(2): 130–8.

Langfield-Smith, K. and Smith, D. (2003) 'Management control systems and trust in outsourcing relationships', *Management accounting research*, 14: 281–307.

Laverack, G. (2005) *Public health – power, empowerment and professional practice.* London: Palgrave Macmillan.

Laverack, G. and Labonte, R. (2000) 'A planning framework for community empowerment goals within health promotion', *Health policy and planning*, 15(3): 255–62.

Lenihan, P. (2005) 'MAPP and the evolution of planning in public health practice', *Public health management practice*, 11(5): 381–6.

Levin, M. (1988) *Lokal mobilisering.* Institutt for industriell miljøforsking. Trondheim: SINTEF-Gruppen.

Lindblom, C. E. (1959) 'The science of "muddling through"', *Public Administration Review*, 19(2): 79–88.

Lindblom, C. E. (1979) 'Still muddling, not yet through', *Public Administration Review*, 39(6): 517–26.

Lukes, S. (1974) *Power: a radical view*. London: Macmillan.

Lundquist, L. (1976) 'Några synspunkter på begreppet politisk planering', *Statsvetenskapleg Tidsskrift*, 79(2): 121–39.

McKenzie, J. F., Neiger, B. L. and Smeltzer, J. L. (2005) *Planning, implementation, and evaluating health promotion programs*. London: Pearson Education. Benjamin Cummings.

Manin, B. (1987) 'On legitimacy and political deliberation', *Political Theory*, 15(3): 338–68.

March, J. G. and Olsen, J. P. (eds) (1976) *Ambiguity and choice in organizations*. Bergen: Universitetsforlaget.

Miller, R. L. and Campbell, R. (2006) 'Taking stock of empowerment evaluation', *American Journal of Evaluation*, 27(3): 296–319.

Minogue, M. (1993) 'Theory and practice in public policy and administration', in M. Hill (ed.) *The policy process. A reader*. London: Harvester Wheatsheaf.

Morgan, G. and Smircich, L. (1980) 'The caser for qualitative research', *Academy of Management Review*, 5(4): 491–500.

Nicola, R. M. and Hatcher, M. T. (2000) 'A framework for building effective public health constituencies', *Public Health Management Practice*, 6(2): 1–10.

Norman, R. (2006) *Managing for outcomes while accounting for outputs. Defining public value in New Zealand's performance management system*. Paper for AESOP Conference. Leuven, Belgium, 1–3 June 2006. Wellington: Victoria University of Wellington.

OECD (2002) *Distributed public governance. Agencies, authorities and other government bodies*. Paris: Organization for Economic Co-operation and Development.

OECD (2003) 'Public sector modernisation', in *Policy brief, October 2003*. Paris: Organization for Economic Co-operation and Development.

Offerdal, A. (1992) *Den politiske kommunen*. Oslo: Det Norske Samlaget.

Olsen, J. P. (1988) *Administrative reforms and theories of organization*. Notat 88/31. Bergen: LOS-senteret.

Olsen, J. P. (2004) *Innovasjon, politikk og institusjonell dynamikk*. Working paper 04/04. University of Oslo: Centre for European Studies.

Østfold County Council (2005) *The HEPRO project plan*. Sarpsborg: Østfold County Council.

Paasi, A. (1986) 'The institutionalization of regions: a theoretical framework for understanding the emergence of regions and the constitution of regional identity', *Fennia*, 164: 105–46.

Paasi, A., Raatikka, A., Raivo, P. and Riikonen, H. (1994) 'Regions, places and landscape: research in regional and human geography at Oulu University', *Fennia*, 172: 153–61.

Pollitt, C. and Bouckaert, G. (2000) *Public management reform: a comparative analysis*. Oxford: University Press.

Prilleltensky, I. (2005) 'Promoting well-being: time for a paradigm shift in health and human services', *Scandinavian Journal of Public Health*, 33: 53–60.

Putnam, R. D. (1993) *Making democracy work: civic traditions in modern Italy*. Princeton, NJ: Princeton University Press.

Rasmussen, N. Kr. and Wangberg, A. (2009) *Eurohepro 2006–2007. Results from six countries in the Baltic Sea region*. Sarpsborg: Østfold County Council. Available at: www.heproforum.net/images/stories/uploads/PDF/Surveys/eurohepro_final.pdf.

Rokkan, S. and Urwin, D. W. (1983) *Economy, territory, identity: politics of West European peripheries*. London: Sage.

Sager, T. (1990) *Communicate or calculate. Planning theory and social science concepts in a contingency perspective*. NORDPLAN dissertation 11. Stockholm: Nordic Institute for Studies in Urban and Regional Planning.

Sager, T. (1992) 'Why plan? A multi-rationality foundation for planning', *Scandinavian Housing & Planning Research*, 9: 129–47.

Salem, E. (2005) 'The promise of MAPP: a transformational tool for public health practice', *Public Health Management Practice*, 11(5): 379–80.

Scambler, G. (ed.) (2001a) *Habermas, critical theory and health*. Florence, KY: Routledge.

Scambler, G. (2001b) 'Unfolding themes of an incomplete project', in *Habermas, critical theory and health*. Florence, KY: Routledge.

Scharpf, F. W. (2001) 'Notes towards a theory of multilevel governing in Europe', *Scandinavian Political Studies*, 24(1): 1–16.

Schön, D. (1983) *The reflective practitioner. How professionals think in action*. London: Temple Smith.

Schön, D. (1986) 'Toward a new epistemology of practice', in B. Checkoway (ed.) *Strategic perspectives of planning practice*. Lexington, MA: Lexington Books.

Schulz, A. J., Israel, B. A., Zimmerman, M. A. and Checkoway, B. N. (1995) 'Empowerment as multi-level construct: perceived control at the individual, organizational, and community level', *Health Education Research*, 10(3): 309–27.

Senge, P. (1990) *The fifth discipline: the art and practice of the learning organization*. New York: Doubleday.

Simon, H. A. (1965) *Administrative man*. Glencoe: Free Press.

Stöhr, W. B. (1990) 'Synthesis', 'Introduction' and 'On the theory and practice of local development in Europe', in W. B. Stöhr (ed.) *Global challenge and local response*. London, New York: Mansell.

Stoker, G. (1997) 'Public–private partnership and urban governance', in G. Stoker (ed.) *Partners in urban governance: European and American experience*. London: Macmillan.

Stoker, G. (1998) 'Governance as theory, five propositions', *Social Science Journal*, 50: 17–28.

Stoker, G. (2004) *Transforming local governance. From Thatcherism to New Labour*. London: Palgrave Macmillan.

Storper, M. (1997) *The regional world: territorial development in a global economy*. New York: Guilford.

Strand, T. (2001) *Ledelse, organizasjon og kultur*. Bergen: Fagbokforlaget.

Svendsen, G. T. and Svendsen, G. L. H. (2006) *Social kapital. En introduktion*. København: Hans Reitzels.

Swyngedouw, E. (2005) 'Governance innovation and the citizen: the Janus face of governance-beyond-the-state', *Urban Studies*, 42(11): 1191–2006.

Tones, K. (1974) 'A systems approach to health education', *Community Health*, 6: 34–9.

Tones, K. and Green, J. (2004) *Health promotion*. London: Sage Publications.

United Nations (2009) *Planning sustainable cities. Global report on human settlements*. United Nations Human Settlements Programme. London, Sterling: Earthscan.

Uyarra, E. (2007) 'Key dilemmas of regional innovation policies', *Innovation*, 20(3): 243–61.

Vega, J. and Irwin, A. (2004) 'Tackling health inequalities: new approaches in public policy', *Bulletin of the World Health Organization*, 82(7): 482–3.

Veggeland, N. (2000) *Den nye regionalismen*. Bergen: Fagbokforlaget.

Wangberg, A. and Dyrseth, T. (eds) (2008) *HEPRO toolkit. A guide to sustainable health planning process*. Sarpsborg: Østfold County Council. Available at: www. heproforum.net/images/stories/uploads/PDF/hepro_toolkit_final.pdf.

WHO (1978) *Declaration of Alma Ata*. Geneva: World Health Organization

WHO (1986) *Ottawa charter for health promotion*. Geneva: World Health Organization.

WHO (1991) *Sundsvall statement on supportive environments for health*. Geneva: World Health Organization.

WHO (1997) *The Jakarta declaration*. Geneva: World Health Organization.

WHO (2001) *Evaluation in health promotion. Principles and perspectives*. WHO regional publications European series, 92. Geneva: World Health Organization.

Wilson, K. (2004) 'The complexities of multi-level governance in public health', *Canadian Journal of Public Health*, 95(6): 409–12.

Zoete, P. R. (2000) *Towards informal levels in urban and regional planning*. Paper presented at the 14th AESOP Congress, Brno, Czech Republic, 18–23 July.

Author index

Subject index